Bread
Is the
Devil

Bread
Is the
Devil

Win the Weight
Loss Battle
by Taking Control
of Your
Diet Demons

Heather Bauer, R.D., C.D.N.,
and Kathy Matthews

St. Martin's Press ☙ New York

This book is intended as a reference volume only, not as a medical manual. The information given here is designed to help you make informed decisions about your health. The dietary programs in this book are not intended as a substitute for any dietary regimen that may have been prescribed by your doctor. You should discuss all new dietary programs with your doctor before beginning.

BREAD IS THE DEVIL. Copyright © 2012 by Heather Bauer. All rights reserved. Printed in the United States of America. For information, address St. Martin's Press, 175 Fifth Avenue, New York, N.Y. 10010.

www.stmartins.com

Library of Congress Cataloging-in-Publication Data

Bauer, Heather.
   Bread is the devil : win the weight loss battle by taking control of your diet demons / Heather Bauer and Kathy Matthews.
       p. cm.
   ISBN 978-1-250-00022-4
   1. Weight loss.   2. Food habits.   I. Matthews, Kathy, 1949–   II. Title.
   RM222.2.B38575 2012
   613.2'5—dc23

                                                                2011035844

First Edition: January 2012

10 9 8 7 6 5 4 3 2 1

To Ross, my everything

Contents

PART 4 Sticking with It

PART 5 Resources

Bread
Is the
Devil

Introduction

Let's face it, everyone knows what goes into losing weight—it's all about eating less and exercising more, right? So why do you (and your best friend and your neighbor and your mother) still struggle with those stubborn pounds?

I can help you because I've been studying diet behavior for eleven years and working with clients who have successfully and permanently reached their weight loss goals. I've come up with a program that works. It's a combination of healthy foods and—here's the difference—behavioral strategies that help you contend with the situations and emotions that prompt you to eat more than you should and more than you even want. I call these triggers Devils. If you've struggled to lose weight, you have at least one Devil, and maybe many more, sitting on your shoulder, making it challenging if not impossible for you to make good decisions when it comes to food.

"I'm good all day, but the moment I walk in the door at five I can't stop eating until I fall into bed."

"I pick, pick, pick all afternoon long: cookies, brownies, crackers, you name it."

"I'm great all week, but the weekends are killers. I just inhale food all weekend."

"I'm almost never hungry, but I eat when I'm tired, when I'm stressed and when I'm bored."

"I eat well at home, but when I eat out I'm a lost cause. And I eat out a lot."

Do any of these people sound like you? If so, you have a Diet Devil on your shoulder and I'm going to help you get rid of it.

The Devils that ruin our diets have this in common: they're situations—foods, people, occasions—that prompt indulgences. These indulgences are never fruits or veggies or protein; they're bagels, muffins, pasta, chips, pizza, cakes, candies and all those poppable, pickable foods that keep me in business and keep *you* struggling to get in your skinny jeans.

Take the Devil I like to call the Late-Night Shuffle—that mindless munching we do in the evening. And then there's travel, or Road Hogging, which blasts our schedules to hell and makes overeating seem like an essential reward. And, oh Lord, for many of us it's children—those small creatures who insist on cookies and waffles and peanut butter, which is in constant supply in your very own kitchen. We all have a Devil or two that keeps us from losing weight successfully. It's in our heads or in our fridges or sometimes it's waiting for us at the airport café when we're delayed and tired and irritable.

Almost all popular diets ignore these Devils under the mistaken belief that telling you what to eat will solve your weight problems. But with your Diet Devils on your shoulder, you'll find—you've probably already found—that no diet is going to work for long. For most people, trying to stick to a typical diet is like trying to learn to ski without an instructor. You can do your best, but chances are you're going to fall down so many times that eventually you'll get discouraged and quit. Yes, diets are hard. And what makes it worse is that we are sick and tired of them.

But when you identify your particular Devils, the whole game changes. It's like having an angel on your shoulder to get you through the rough patches. Banish your Diet Devils and weight loss becomes doable. Not always easy. No one would claim that. But very possible. And permanent.

Strategic Eating

When it comes to bad food choices, it's not that we don't know better. Nobody thinks that downing a sleeve of Ritz crackers with peanut butter while watching the Academy Awards is a good diet choice. Nobody thinks that distracting a toddler so you can filch their McDonald's fries is a good diet choice. *People are not clueless about what to eat.* But most are vulnerable to one or more Devils that prompt them to eat too much and too often.

The Diet Devils turn people into Situational Eaters. What's a Situational Eater? Perhaps you've heard of the seefood diet? You see food, you eat it. A Situational Eater listens to the Devil on her shoulder and lets the environment dictate what and how much she eats. Those bedeviled Situational Eaters are often not even hungry. Sometimes they're not even tasting the food; they're feeding an emotion or they're bored or distracted: they're victims of their Diet Devils.

Here's an example: Many of my clients report that they abandoned a diet when they experienced the Plunge. The Plunge is one of the Diet Devils that's so common that many people spend a lifetime victimized by it. A typical Plunge goes something like this: You've been eating clean for a week. You can easily button your pants. But now it's the weekend and you have so much to catch up on. As you rush through the supermarket, tossing things in your cart, you find yourself grabbing a bag of cheddar popcorn. For your son. Or your husband, you tell yourself. But by the time you're halfway home, you're a quarter of the way through that bag of popcorn. You feel kind of queasy; definitely not good. And you're not hungry for dinner so you just have a few chunks of cheese. And then two bowls of cereal. Make that three. And now, feeling like you've ruined your week, you sink into the sofa with a big goblet of wine. You say to yourself, "What's the point?" And that's the Plunge. And that's the end of that diet. And now you're more demoralized and defeated than ever.

A Strategic Eater, on the other hand, has a set of premade decisions and strategies, so when the environment says, "sourdough," the Strategic Eater says, "*mais non!*" Once you become a Strategic Eater, you'll be master of your food universe, master of your Devils. When you're tempted, instead of blundering along mindlessly, you'll be able to pause and say, "Wait . . . I've seen this movie and I know how it ends." You'll be able to rewrite your script.

Diet Devils: The Inspiration for *Bread Is the Devil*

When I first began to work with clients who needed help losing weight, I quickly realized that a formal diet wasn't going to be the solution. For one thing, I had a very particular type of client who tended to be somewhat "diet resistant," even if they told me that they wanted to lose weight. Because I drew many of my clients from a downtown New York City gym that offered their members free consultations with me, many of these people were high-powered workers who were looking for fast results and were resistant to making lots of changes in their demanding lifestyles. Most of them wanted to lose weight but they were skeptical that it would actually happen. They were too busy. They ate out a lot. They didn't really have much time to exercise. They traveled, etc., etc. They only came to see me because it was free. Talking to these people about good nutrition and sensible food plans was pretty much like trying to teach kittens to fly. I knew I needed a totally different approach if I was going to achieve success with them and build my business. So I began to work backward when looking for solutions to weight gain. When my clients came to see me, I asked them to fill out a form that included a question about any diets they'd tried in the past. After the first few clients, I revised the form to allow for more space for the answer to this question. Most of my clients had been on at least three diets and often more. I soon realized that this pattern would lead me to the crucial question that would be the key to their diet success. Why did they fail at a diet? What situation or habit or event caused them to either abandon a diet or overeat? The answer to this question became the Diet Devils.

Surprisingly, most people have never thought about the reasons for their diet failures, no matter how many diets they've been on. Most people assume that "the diet didn't work for me" (the magic of weird body chemistry), or they blame their "lack of willpower" or boredom with the diet itself. But when asked for a particular reason that they fell off a particular diet, most clients can identify one or two Devils that had knocked them off their diet track, whether it was a vacation or a dinner party or extreme work or family stress or perhaps something as simple as a single "forbidden" slice of pizza that cascaded into a massive failure of control.

I now know without a doubt that helping people recognize and tame their Diet Devils while simultaneously guiding them to healthy, appropriate eating patterns is the most effective way for them to achieve permanent weight loss.

In the Beginning: Lessons of the Zamboni

I'm probably a lot like you when it comes to struggles with eating. Even though I've never really been overweight (good genes;

lots of exercise; knowing my Devils intimately), I struggle to eat well and stay on track most every day. A lot of what I know about weight control I learned from my own experience. I really know what I'm talking about when it comes to Diet Devils. I've been there. I think my clients realize this as soon as they meet me. I'm not one of those skinny nutritionists who say, "Stop eating when you're full" and "Avoid snacks" and "Eliminate alcohol." I know that for many of us these simple rules just don't work. We need clever strategies and clever advance planning to reach our goals.

Here's a story that will demonstrate why I understand the Late-Night Shuffle, the Plunge and all the Devils I describe in this book:

Shortly after I met my husband, Ross, I visited my family in Maryland, gushing about this great guy who could just be my Mr. Right. "And guess what he calls me?" I announced. "His little Zamboni!"

My brother's jaw dropped. "Heather, do you know what a Zamboni is?"

"Well, I guess it's some kind of Italian endearment or something. I know his family visits Italy a lot."

"Heather," my brother explained over the growing laughter, "a Zamboni is that thing that cleans up the ice after a hockey game. He's calling you an eating machine, and I bet it has something to do with your blazing eating speed."

What can I say? I grew up in Maryland, with no experience of hockey or ice rinks. And the truth is, I am a Zamboni. Always have been. I love to eat. Sometimes, when not paying attention, I eat like the gun just went off in a food race.

It was my Zamboni-like inclinations that forced me to become a Strategic Eater at an early age. If I followed my natural inclinations, I could sub for a float in the Macy's Thanksgiving Day Parade.

Here's the important point I'm trying to make: I recognize

and accept the type of eater I am. I'm just not the kind of girl who can open a pint of ice cream without finishing it. I'll never be the girl who can eat one piece of bread from the breadbasket. My message to all you food fighters out there: stop fighting it. Accept the type of eater you are, learn the strategies that work for you and learn to recover when you fall off track.

This book is a guide for all those Zambonis who are tired of fighting their own inclinations. Tired of playing Whac-a-Mole with every food temptation that makes losing ten or twenty pounds or more seem impossible. This is a guide for everyone who's lost the patience to read one more diet book. Who doesn't want to follow a strict eating plan or eat "fake" food. Who isn't into complicated systems or gimmicks or short-term results.

A Note About the Title

Even though *Bread Is the Devil* is my title, this is not another low-carb diet book. I don't believe in banishing carbs, because our bodies need them—the good kind, anyway. There are good carbs such as beans and whole grains, and then there are bad, or what I call Devil, carbs, like cookies, candy, and white bread. It's the Devil Carbs that get us in trouble.

Many of us have been there: a sensible, healthy breakfast, high in protein with complex carbs. Ditto for lunch—soup and a salad with a warm rush of accomplishment and self-control for dessert. And now it's dinnertime and you're out with friends. The waiter sets a large basket of warm, sliced, crusty sourdough on the table with a little plate of chive butter. And suddenly you're in the seventh circle of hell. The breadbasket is empty. Your lap is full of crumbs and the bread IS the devil. The phrase is shorthand for the inevitable, demonic pull that certain bad habits exert on us. That's why *Bread Is the Devil*. But my simple, balanced, healthy-eating plan plus my innovative, effective behavorial strategies will help you banish bread and all the other Devils.

How to Use This Book

There are five parts to this book:

1. Unmasking Your Diet Devils

2. The Blueprint

3. Taming Your Diet Devils

4. Sticking with It

5. Resources

In "Unmasking Your Diet Devils," I'll introduce the ten Devils and you'll take a simple quiz that will help you identify your own Devil (or Devils!). You'll also learn how to create a food journal that will serve as an effective tool in guiding you to permanent weight loss.

The second part of the book outlines the Blueprint, the twenty-one-day, step-by-step, day-by-day guide for what to eat and how much. (The Blueprint covers your first twenty-one days of my diet because research shows that it takes that long—twenty-one days—to change a habit.) Now, some of my clients pull a big frowny face when I start to pull out my Blueprint. *Until they read it.* It's so simple and easy to remember. In addition to the eating plan, the Blueprint provides specific advice that will help you on your way, such as how to adjust the eating plan to suit your weight loss goals. And it will tell you how to deal with plateaus and how to live with my plan once you do reach your goal weight. And, by the way, it's important that you commit to those first twenty-one days of the Blueprint. This will give you time to really see progress. We all lose weight at different rates. Some lucky people will drop five pounds in a week. But it's much more common for weight loss to be erratic. I've had many clients who stay the same weight for ten days or fifteen days and then suddenly, for no reason anyone can point to, they begin to drop pounds. I've seen it countless times: Clients who stick to the Blueprint for twenty-one days lose weight. So be patient: Commit to the twenty-one days. You will see weight loss and it will last a lifetime.

The third part of the book, "Taming Your Diet Devils," provides simple, effective strategies that will help you manage permanent weight loss. In this section you will learn more about your particular Devils and how to eliminate their influence. This is the personalized part of the book: You'll be learning strategies that apply directly to your life, and these strategies will help you eliminate or avoid the situations that used to be your diet downfalls. You'll be sticking to your diet and losing weight for real in no time.

The fourth part, "Sticking with It," will answer your questions about how to handle plateaus, maintenance, and other issues that might crop up as you continue with the diet.

In the fifth and last section, "Resources," I include a restaurant guide that you'll find indispensible if you enjoy eating out and a terrific shopping guide with my favorite foods as well as some recipes and cooking tips.

Now let's get started.

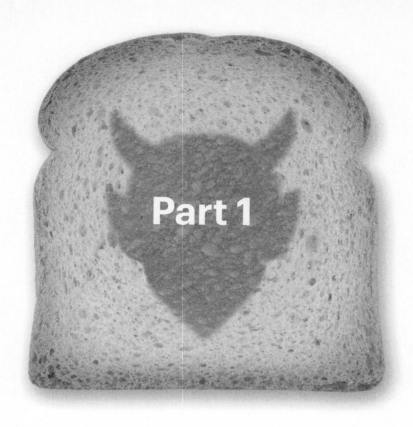

Part 1

Unmasking
Your Diet Devils

When I meet a client in my office for the first time, I become a diet detective. My job is to try and figure out why this person can't lose weight. Most people come to me having done a host of diets, pills, shakes, cleanses, hypnotherapy, diet spas, ashram visits . . . you name it. So I begin asking questions. What's going on in your life? Are you single? Married? A workaholic? A commuter? Do you have kids? Live alone? Which diet worked best for you in the past? This last question tells me if you can eat carbs or if carbs are a trigger, and if portion control is an issue for you or if it's more about food choices. Every answer brings me closer to understanding what has held you back in the past. By the end of the session I know why you can't lose weight or can't lose enough weight, or why you lost weight and then gained it back. Now I know your Devils and I know how to guide you to permanent weight loss.

Permanent weight loss is not just about what you eat—it's about behavior. We all know what to eat. *It's the behavior that's hard to change.* That's why I find my clients have great success when they work with a relatively flexible eating plan while focusing on the circumstances—the Devils—that prompt them to eat. You most likely know what to eat. But it's those moments of weakness, stress or boredom you need help with: your night eating, your picking morsels off your kids' plates, your candy grabs at the receptionist's desk, your struggle with eating out without pigging out and all the other Devils that throw you off track.

So what Diet Devils do you have? Below are a series of questions I ask my clients when I am trying to determine what gets them off track. A number that refers to one of the ten Devils follows each question (in a few instances, there is more than one Devil identified). Go through and answer the questions, and jot down the numbers that apply to you. After the quiz, review your numbers—the numbers that show up most frequently are your major Devils—and see which Devils you need to concentrate on.

The Devil Detective Quiz

Are there certain people in your life who trigger you to eat unhealthy foods?	☑ Yes	☐ No	(4)
Do you usually eat everything on your plate?	☑ Yes	☐ No	(2)
Have you tried and failed at more than one diet?	☑ Yes	☐ No	(1)
Do you eat quickly?	☑ Yes	☐ No	(2, 10)
Do you have a secret stash of snacks in your desk drawer?	☐ Yes	☑ No	(6)
If you open a bag of chips, are you pretty sure to empty it?	☐ Yes	☑ No	(2)
Do you tend to lose weight when you're on vacation?	☐ Yes	☑ No	(6)
Are you a heat-seeking missile for a waiter with a tray of crab puffs?	☐ Yes	☑ No	(8)

Are you still holding on to your pregnancy weight even though your child is taking his SATs?	☑ Yes	☐ No	(5)
Do you eat well during the week and blow it on weekends?	☑ Yes	☐ No	(6)
Is nighttime snack time for you?	☐ Yes	☑ No	(3)
Do you think a trip to the supermarket is exercise?	☐ Yes	☑ No	(7)
Do you like airline food?	☐ Yes	☑ No	(9)
Do you find competitive moms drive you right to the ice cream for comfort?	☐ Yes	☑ No	(5, 4)
Do you regularly indulge in Mish-Mosh dinners (a bowl of cereal, a cup of yogurt and a spoonful of peanut butter)?	☐ Yes	☑ No	(6, 1, 5)
Do you find that one diet "mistake" or binge will throw you completely off track?	☑ Yes	☐ No	(2)
Do you eat out more than twice a week?	☑ Yes	☐ No	(10)
Do you eat healthier when you exercise?	☑ Yes	☐ No	(4, 7)
Are you capable of stealing a child's Halloween candy?	☑ Yes	☐ No	(5)
Do you find it hard to eat well on weekends?	☑ Yes	☐ No	(6)
Does drinking (alcohol) trigger you to make worse food choices at that meal or the day after you drink?	☑ Yes	☐ No	(8, 10)
Is your mood affected by how well you eat?	☑ Yes	☐ No	(4)
Have you ever eaten a french fry from your kid's car seat?	☐ Yes	☑ No	(5)
Can you stop at just twelve almonds?	☑ Yes	☐ No	(2)

Do you tend to gain weight while traveling (even if your destination is just an outlet mall)?	☑ Yes	☐ No	(9)
Have you noticed that certain foods—perhaps sugar, salt or bread—are triggers for you?	☑ Yes	☐ No	(2)
Do you "wing it" when trying to lose weight, with no particular plan? Do you tend to say to yourself, "I really should lose some weight" without taking any action?	☑ Yes	☐ No	(1)
Do you tend to eat more when you are alone?	☐ Yes	☑ No	(6, 3)
Do you eat things you really don't want to please others or to "fit in"?	☐ Yes	☑ No	(4)
Do you skip breakfast in the morning because you aren't hungry?	☐ Yes	☑ No	(3)
Did you use to exercise while in college but no longer do?	☑ Yes	☐ No	(7)
Do you entertain a lot for work?	☐ Yes	☑ No	(10)
Do you gain weight at holiday time—November to January?	☑ Yes	☐ No	(8)
Do you find it hard to eat well when you go home to visit your parents or relatives?	☑ Yes	☐ No	(8)
Do you spend a lot of time in your car, commuting, doing errands or traveling to a weekend house?	☐ Yes	☑ No	(9)
Are you likely to eat when angry, frustrated or sad?	☑ Yes	☐ No	(4)

The Answer Key: Introducing the Ten Devils

If the same number pops up for you multiple times, this is your main Devil that throws you off your diet track. If you wrote down more than one number, you have a few Devils troubling you. Here is a brief description of each Devil:

1. **FREE-STYLE DIETING.** This is the Devil that prompts you to try to lose weight on your own—no plan, no real strategy, no serious commitment, just the hope that cutting down on your food intake or eliminating a category of food or promising yourself "no more cookies" will have the desired effect. If you've tried this approach, you're not alone and you no doubt know that it just doesn't work. You typically find yourself right back where you started when life throws you a curveball—or a giant meatball. After a Free-Style failure, you're typically more discouraged than ever. Well, banish your half-hearted stab at dieting. My Free-Style strategies will convince you to commit to a plan and thus lose the weight once and for all. Once you've banished the Free-Style Devil, your head will be in the right diet space and you'll be empowered to adopt your new healthy-eating lifestyle. *(See page 79.)*

2. **THE PLUNGE.** This is the Devil that prompts you to true despair. It's the uncontrolled binge, often after a stretch of successful dieting. It's a pint of Ben & Jerry's or an entire sleeve of chocolate chip cookies or all of the above. It makes you feel hopeless and totally out of control. Almost all of my clients have suffered the Plunge, and it usually throws them completely off track. You may be surprised by my basic approach to a Plunge: I believe the most important strategy for Plungers is not trying

to forever ban a Plunge. That may not be possible. Rather the strategies I outline for Plungers help them to navigate the dark waters of binge eating by not only learning to recognize and avoid temptations to the Plunge but also, more important, learning to recover from a Plunge and go on. It's only partly about the actual eating: More critical is what goes on in your mind post-Plunge. My strategies will help you recover from a Plunge and move on to renewed efforts and ultimate success. *(See page 87.)*

3. **THE LATE-NIGHT SHUFFLE.** It could be a bag of popcorn, a box of crackers, a series of frozen treats but, really, what it's about is a bad habit. It's the routine of nighttime, after-dinner snacking that has perhaps become a part of your daily routine. You vow each morning that you'll never do it again, but without the right strategies it's a losing battle. Many people are unaware of how these evening calories can add up. They can eat well all day but somehow ignore the morsels they consume come sundown. Some people rely on "diet" snacks in the evening, but these can be as counterproductive as any other munchies. It's not terribly difficult to banish the Late-Night Shuffle. You just need to recognize the habit and use my strategies to substitute good behaviors for bad. Once you achieve this, you'll be amazed at the effect it has on your weight loss progress. *(See page 99.)*

4. **EMOTIONAL EATING.** This is the Devil that lodges snugly in your head. It's not about hunger; it's not about habit. It's about how you feel and how that makes you eat. An overheard criticism of your parenting skills? A boss who's piling on the work until you're so stressed your hair is falling out? A relative who prods you to

overeat at each holiday meal? Emotions are powerful, and if you don't recognize how they can sabotage your diet it's almost impossible to win the battle with this Devil. I'll outline the issues that could prompt you to be an Emotional Eater and, more important, the simple strategies that will help you recognize Emotional Eating and avoid it in the future. *(See page 113.)*

5. **LITTLE DEVILS.** We all adore our children, but they can make it hard to lose weight in so many little devilish ways, from the time they steal from our exercise routines to the tempting foods they eat, like peanut butter and Halloween treats. It's challenging to eat lean and clean when you're trying to satisfy their growing bodies. But it's not impossible. I'll show you how to eat well whether you're dealing with the common "double dinner" dilemma of parenting (one with daddy; one with the kids) or the post–soccer practice, fast-food challenge. I even have strategies for dealing with picky eaters and the challenge of feeding the "skinny kid" as well as the delicate issue of little girls who are watching Mommy diet. *(See page 130.)*

6. **BOREDOM BINGEING.** Eating is fun. It's pleasurable. It's a tempting way to fill an empty afternoon. But there's a big price to pay. Many of us don't recognize that Boredom Bingeing can add hundreds of calories to our daily intake and can make permanent weight loss near impossible. Boredom Bingeing is all about mindless eating. Snacking, munching, noshing, nibbling. . . . Not because you're hungry or because you're sitting at an actual meal but because you're faced with a bowl of candy or someone left muffins in the office kitchen or you are simply trying to fill an empty niche in your day by checking the fridge one more time. Boredom

Bingeing is distracted eating. It's not really pleasurable or satisfying. Why do we eat when we're not really hungry? Same reason people climb mountains: because they're there. You can break yourself of Boredom Bingeing and get a real boost in your weight loss progress, as well as a real boost to your self-esteem, by using my Boredom Bingeing strategies and getting better control of your time as well as your eating. I'll teach you how to regulate your meals so you'll stay satisfied and thus better control your food intake and banish Boredom Bingeing forever. *(See page 145.)*

7. **SLOTH.** This Devil is about exercising, or rather, *not* exercising. It's the "don't get out of your chair, your favorite program is coming on" Devil. But moving more is important to weight loss. It's not *the* most important factor, but it definitely plays a role, and I'll show you how you can tame the Sloth Devil and turbocharge your weight loss. Some clients are nervous when they come to see me because they don't exercise and they feel guilty about it. If this is you, relax. When you deal with your Sloth Devil, I firmly believe that managing your food intake is the first and most important step you can take to lose weight. You're going to work on that goal first. And then, when you're ready, I'll show you some very simple strategies that will help you work exercise into your schedule. You may surprise yourself and become a marathoner. But even if you simply add some regular activity to your life, I'll show you how getting off the sofa is going to make a big difference to your long-term health and weight. *(See page 161.)*

8. **CELEBRATIONS! VACATIONS!** Nothing's more fun than a party or a trip, but too often these events totally derail our best diet intentions. Whether it's an office

holiday party, a cousin's wedding or your long-awaited
week at the beach, this Devil prompts us to throw
caution to the wind and indulge, indulge, indulge! So
many people begin a diet and then something comes up:
an anniversary, a trip, a wedding. . . . All their progress
and resolutions go to hell as they slip back into old
habits following a major celebratory indulgence. Life
doesn't have to be like this. It really is possible to
manage special events without losing control. Whether
you're heading out of the country on a dream trip to
Paris or simply trying to cope with an upcoming dinner
party, I have the techniques that will help you eat well.
Sometimes it's a matter of knowing how to *think* about
eating while on vacation. Other times it's navigating an
office birthday party. No matter: If this is your Devil,
I'll show you how to eat well and have fun at the same
time. *(See page 175.)*

9. **ROAD HOGGING.** This is the devil that sits on your
   dashboard. Or in your carry-on bag. Or anywhere you
   travel. It knocks you off your schedule and lures you into
   making excuses for poor food choices and erratic eating.
   It's really a challenge to eat well while traveling, whether
   you're doing your daily commute or flying around the
   world on business. It's difficult to deal with delayed
   meals, canceled meals and food that you'd never choose if
   you had a choice. If RoadHogging bedevils you, I can
   help. I have solutions to the road-food blues and tips that
   can help you navigate every conveyance from a plane to a
   minivan. You can manage a healthy, satisfying airport
   breakfast as well as an easy posttrip reentry dinner with
   the RoadHogging strategies. *(See page 195.)*

10. **THE DINE-OUT DEVIL.** Dine-Out Devils are one of the
    most common dilemmas faced by my clients. Do you eat

out frequently? Eating well at restaurants is a special challenge. If you dine out regularly for business or pleasure, you need help in navigating restaurant menus—and alcohol choices—so that you can reach your weight loss goals. The simple fact is that eating out can be fraught with diet pitfalls—beginning with the bread that lands on the table the minute you sit down. But there's good news on the restaurant scene these days: Chefs are working hard to satisfy the desire many people have to eat well and to limit their calorie intake. Of course you do need some tricks and strategies if you're going to enjoy restaurant food and lose weight at the same time. I will help you with everything from how to navigate a fast-food restaurant to how to manage alcohol while sticking to your weight loss goals. I have simple "restaurant rules" that will make eating out and losing weight mutually compatible. *(See page 214.)*

Now that you have identified your Diet Devils, let's see how we can conquer them!

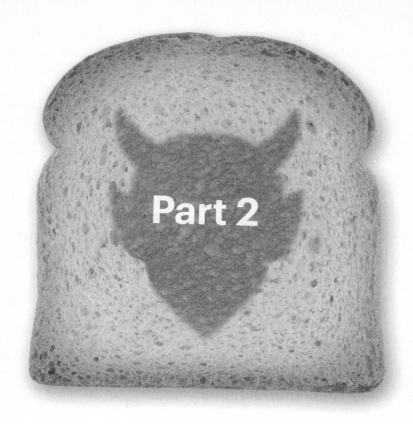

Part 2

The Blueprint

We all know that losing weight is not rocket science. It's just food. Eat less and focus on cleaner food, less junk, more fiber, protein, fruit, veggies so you stay fuller longer and eat less between meals and at meals. But you definitely need guidance—a system—that will help you choose the best food in any situation and avoid those Diet Devils. So I've created a unique and very simple eating plan that guides people to their goal. I call it the Blueprint. I learned early on from my clients that any eating plan that was rigid in its food choices would not work because those plans flew out the window when one of the Diet Devils showed up. Too many people told me how they gained back weight they'd lost after the birth of a baby or taking on a job that required entertaining or enjoying a wedding or party that led them to indulge. So I've created a plan that's simple, flexible, and easy to remember and stick with.

This plan allows you to live—to eat out, to enjoy snacks, even to grab a fast-food restaurant meal with your kids. As I said in the introduction, the Blueprint is the first part of what makes my diet work. When you combine it with the strategies that apply to your particular Devil (which you will read later in the book), you *will* meet your weight loss goal. Almost all my clients have told me that the Blueprint changed the way they thought about dieting and helped them make easy choices in every dining situation. They appreciate that the Blueprint, along with the strategies to conquer their Devils, is all they need to lose weight. And just like them, you're going to say, "I can do this."

Bread Is the Devil Diet in a nutshell:

Identify your Devils (page 11).

Read the Blueprint chart (page 23).

Check out my sample menus for meal ideas (page 48).

Write down menu ideas for breakfast, lunch, snack and dinner.

Create your shopping list and buy your essentials (page 62).

Each week jot down three to five goals in your food journal (e.g., no Devil Carbs, more water).

Record what you eat in your food journal (page 68).

Review your Devils and your strategies.

Remember the power of twenty-one days!

Let's take a bird's-eye look at my Blueprint Chart, which outlines my unique approach to weight loss. You'll see it has three columns. The first column lists all the food categories— from carbs to vegetables to condiments to snacks—that you need to consider in making food choices. You'll see that my categories are not the categories you'd find in a traditional food pyramid. Rather I like to just focus on the food areas that demand daily attention, like beverages and fiber and snacks, categories that most diets ignore but that play a big role in promoting fast weight loss. By dividing the world of food into these categories, I make it extremely easy for you to be flexible in your food choices and also to avoid the foods that lead to weight gain. The second column in the chart designates what amount of the listed food I recommend. The third column lists particular foods in that category.

The Blueprint Chart

Category	Recommended Amount	Particulars
Devil Carbs	Zero	White bread, bagels, muffins, scones, candy, bread in the breadbasket, pizza, ice cream, brownies, Danish, pasta
Angel Carbs	1–2 allowed per day	**The familiar Angel Carbs:** brown rice, couscous, quinoa, farro, grains, baked sweet or white potato, sushi roll (1 Angel Carb) **The bready Angel Carbs:** 2 slices light whole wheat bread, 1 Sahara pita; 1 light whole wheat English muffin **The surprising veggie Angel Carbs:** butternut, winter and spaghetti squash, beans, peas, corn **The Angel Carb sauces:** marinara, teriyaki, barbeque, black bean, any sweet sauce or "I don't know what's in it" sauce in a restaurant **The wild card Angel Carb:** any *BID*-approved frozen meal (1 Angel Carb)
Fiber	1–2 servings a day	Crackers: 4–6 FiberRich Bran Crackers or GG Scandinavian Bran Crispsbread (1 serving of fiber)

Category	Recommended Amount	Particulars
		Cereal: ½ cup oatmeal or ½ cup all bran or ¾ cup of Kashi Go Lean
		Gluten-free options: 4 Health Valley Rice Bran Crackers or Mary's Gone Crackers and ¾ cup Mesa Sunrise cereal
Fruits	Up to 3 per day	Apple, ½ cup blueberries, 1 cup cantaloupe, ½ grapefruit, ½ banana, 2 clementines, ½ cup honeydew, 1 orange, 1 peach, 1 plum, 1 cup pineapple, 1 cup raspberries or strawberries, 12 cherries, 17 grapes (1 serving of fruit)
Vegetables	Unlimited (steamed at home; sautéed or steamed when dining out)	Artichoke hearts, asparagus, broccoli, cabbage, carrots, cauliflower, celery, chard, cucumbers, eggplant, escarole, fennel, green beans, green onions, kale, lettuce, mushrooms, peppers, spinach, sprouts, tomatoes, zucchini
Protein	At every meal (baked, broiled, steamed, grilled or poached)	Breakfast: 4–6 egg whites, 1–2 eggs (limit to 5 whole eggs per week), ½ cup cottage cheese, 2 slices of turkey or Canadian bacon, 6–8 ounces low-fat yogurt, 1 packet or 1 scoop protein shake or powder, 1.5 T peanut butter

Category	Recommended Amount	Particulars
		Lunch or dinner (serving is 3 ounces; shoot for 1–2 servings): turkey, chicken, fish, shellfish, lamb, lean sirloin, buffalo, tofu, meat substitutes (check label for serving); vegetarians can choose any bean as a protein.
		Miscellaneous: 8 ounces skim milk, 12 almonds, 1–2 Mini Babybel Light or any Laughing Cow light cheese, 1 serving of shredded light cheese for cooking, ¼ lb bag of fresh sliced turkey
		(1 serving of protein)
Beverages	64 ounces of water per day; no juice or regular soda	Water, seltzer, herbal or green tea
Alcohol	One free drink allowed; a second counts as an Angel Carb	Light beer, wine, vodka or scotch
Fats and oils	Limit	Olive oil, avocado, canola oil, flax seed oil, lite mayonnaise, light salad dressings
Condiments	Use sparingly	Choose: Mustard, balsamic vinegar, salsa, spices, lite soy sauce, seasonings

Category	Recommended Amount	Particulars
		Limit: Sugary salad dressings (e.g., honey mustard, raspberry vinaigrette) and creamy salad dressings See **Angel Carb Sauces**
Snack	Less then 200 calories, low in fat, high in fiber and may have added protein; eaten between lunch and dinner	**Snacks bars:** Kind, Luna, Gnu **Healthy chips:** 1.3 ounce bag of Glenny's soy crisps **Other types:** 2 FiberRich, 1–2 Laughing Cow light cheese or piece of fruit plus string cheese

Note on the Blueprint Chart: My shopping list (page 62) follows the format of my Blueprint: You will find each category of food with a complete listing of the choices in that category there, making it easy for you to shop and easy to vary your dining choices.

> **Your Primary Beginning Diet Goals:**
>
> Eliminate Devil Carbs
> Reduce Angel Carbs!

Understanding the Blueprint

DEVIL CARBS My clients are more confused about carbs than just about any topic having to do with food. It's easy to understand why: There are "good carbs" (whole wheat bread, beans, etc.) and "bad carbs" (pizza, candy, pastry, etc.). And to make things even more confusing, there are also "low-carb" diets, which were all the rage for a while.

So what the heck is the story on carbs? Well, it's actually fairly simple. I've divided carbs into two categories: Devil Carbs and Angel Carbs. Devil Carbs include white bread, white pasta, bagels, muffins, scones, brownies, pretzels, chips, popcorn, Danish, cake, candy, pizza and ice cream. These carbs are to be avoided like, well, the devil! They make your blood sugar spike, your insulin surge in an effort to reduce that sugar in your blood, and then, kaboom, it all collapses like a popped balloon as your blood sugar falls and you feel tired and lethargic. You know this feeling: It's the afternoon "must have coffee; must have cookies; must take nap" feeling that can send you into a spiral of bad food choices, most particularly the Plunge. Some of the people who come to me for help have been munching on Devil Carbs all day long! *Reducing these Devil Carbs is the single most important step you can take to move quickly toward your weight loss goals.* Devil Carbs seem to stimulate your appetite and make you hungry all day; moreover, they have no nutritional value. If it weren't for the bagels, muffins, scones, pasta, pizza, candy and sweets I'd be out of business!

➤ You can have zero Devil Carbs daily.

ANGEL CARBS I make the concept of good carbs easy by creating my own category: Angel Carbs. Angel Carbs are your friends. They keep you full, keep your blood sugar steady, provide lots of nutritional benefits and sit on your shoulder whispering encouragement in your ear. Many people come to me having eliminated carbs entirely from their diet, but I believe that this approach almost guarantees diet failure. When you eliminate a whole category of food from your diet, especially one that's nutritionally significant, you've set yourself up for trouble.

Trigger Foods

If you like to pop it, pick it, dip it, then it's poppable, pickable, dipable and, most important, it's nonstoppable! And any food that's "nonstoppable" for you should be considered a Devil Carb. Any food that can set you off, from high-fiber cereal to oat bran pretzels, to hummus, wasabi peas, cheese, nuts, olives, pickles, dried fruit, grapes—even cherry tomatoes and carrots, which are healthy—should be considered Devil foods. If you can't control yourself around a particular food, even if it's the healthiest food in the world, then cut it out, at least for a while. I suggest you add any personal Devil Foods to the existing Devil Carb list on the Blueprint Chart.

How many Devil Carbs can you eat daily when trying to lose weight? None! With a single exception: If you're ever in a social situation where it's rude not to eat a Devil Carb—say you're at a dinner party and they're serving a special pasta dish, go right ahead and eat. Make it a reasonable portion, record it in your food journal and move on. It's never worth creating a social fuss in order to stick to your diet! Same thing if you're in a business situation where there's nothing but Devil Carbs: Eat a small portion and move on.

Because there's so much confusion about carbs, particularly good carbs, I've broken down my Angel Carbs into five groups to make it easy for you to recognize and remember them: familiar (brown rice, etc.), bready (bread that you can enjoy on the diet), surprising veggie (the carbs that everyone gets particularly confused about, like beans and starchy veggies), sauces (like teriyaki and barbeque sauce which needs attention if you're trying to lose weight) and wild card (frozen dinners, which I talk about in greater detail later in this chapter).

You can enjoy one to two Angel Carbs a day. Counting your

Angel Carbs provides structure to your weekly diet and encourages you to pay attention to your healthy food intake. If you're a veteran dieter whose weight has gone up and down over the years, you will be more successful if you shoot for just one Angel Carb a day. If you have quite a lot of weight to lose or are a big or active man, you can choose more. It's best to try to spread your Angel Carbs throughout the week, but if you're in a situation where you have two or more in one day, just count them and spread the rest through the course of the week. Some of my clients prefer to stick to one Angel Carb daily and up it to two on weekends. One caveat on Angel Carbs: They can't be "stockpiled." In other words, you can't skip Angel Carbs on three days and then have six in one day! Finally, I think it's important to have your Angel Carbs at either lunch or dinner, not at breakfast.

Did you notice that you can eat bread on this diet? Yes, bread is an Angel Carb. And here are the simple bread rules: You can only have bread in a sandwich. This makes it finite. When you're eating out, the bread must be whole wheat or rye; when at home you can choose one of the bread options listed on the shopping list. But how can there be bread on a diet called Bread Is the Devil? Simple. *Whole wheat bread* that's high in fiber, eaten in moderation, is good for you. It's an Angel Carb. Not only does it provide important nutrients, it also fills you up and keeps you satisfied. And, most important, I found that when people can enjoy bread (within certain guidelines), it adds tremendous flexibility to their lives and promotes weight loss success. Sandwiches are readily available most anywhere and my recommended sandwiches—turkey on whole wheat with mustard and lettuce, for example—are typically lower in calories and volume than many salads.

You'll notice that I include frozen dinners as wild card Angel Carbs. Counting them as Angel Carbs simplifies dieters' lives and that's why they're in this category. Choose your frozen dinners from my shopping list. The entire frozen dinner counts as an Angel Carb.

And, finally, if you're a vegetarian, you can count beans as a protein rather than an Angel Carb.

> ➤ You can have 1–2 Angel Carbs daily at lunch or dinner, but none at breakfast.

FIBER, FIBER, FIBER!   Most people think of fiber, well . . . actually, most people don't think much about fiber at all. And if you're trying to lose weight, that's not good. Fiber is rarely listed as a separate category of food, but I found with my clients that it's really effective to count fiber in your weekly food plan. Fiber helps you lose weight by making you feel full. It keeps your system "moving"; it's heart healthy and it stabilizes your blood sugar. Most of us are starving for fiber. The USDA tells us that 80 percent of us don't get enough, and I bet that percentage is even higher among dieters because many sources of fiber are limited on many weight loss plans. Moreover, many people are so mixed up about the most common source of fiber—carbs—that they skip them entirely. And—an important consideration—fiber can provide the satisfying, chewiness we often miss when we're trying to cut down on calories. It really can be a secret weapon in your battle of the bulge.

I recommend two brands of fiber crackers that help you get all the fiber you need: first, the insanely popular FiberRich crackers.[1] Four to six FiberRich crackers equal one serving of fiber—a perfect afternoon snack that keeps you full, keeps you regular and keeps you from overeating at dinner. There's also the popular GG Bran Crispbread crackers, which look and

---

1 See gluten-free options on my Shopping List, page 62, for fiber choices as well as other gluten-free foods.

taste something like roofing tiles but are marvelously crunchy, super high in fiber and can be enjoyed with one of my recommended cheeses for a hunger-banishing snack. The other fiber choices include oatmeal and a selection of high-fiber cereals like Kashi Go Lean.

Remember to keep up with your water consumption when you introduce additional fiber into your diet. If your diet has previously been low in fiber, you may find yourself constipated if you add additional fiber without simultaneously increasing your water intake.

How many fiber choices can you have daily? One to two. That means you can have a nice cereal in the morning, some crispy crumbled FiberRich crackers on your soup or salad at lunch and maybe GG crackers with a recommended cheese in the afternoon. These fiber choices do not count as carbs; just fiber.

➤ You can have 1–2 fibers daily.

FRUIT Some of my clients lived in fear of fruit—all that deathly sugar!—before they came to see me. I don't know how people get such crazy ideas about food! Fruit, in reasonable amounts, is good for you. Fruit provides an abundance of nutrients, natural sweetness and great flavor. I recommend choosing up to three fruits a day. For most people, what I call a "hand fruit"—one that fits in your palm—is a good choice. Hand fruits include apples, peaches, oranges, pears, plums, nectarines or small bananas. Don't forget about frozen fruit. There are great, no-sweetener-added frozen fruits available these days. You can have up to one cup of frozen fruit; check the bag of fruit for specifics. Also, no dried fruit or fruit juice. It's best not to go over your limit of three fruits daily, but if you're really hungry, a piece of fruit is a good choice even if it bumps you over your limit.

➤ You can have up to 3 fruits daily.

VEGETABLES   Oh boy, vegetables! Chow down! You can have unlimited vegetables. I've never, ever had a client who binges on asparagus. And veggies are packed with important nutrients as well as fiber. So go to town.

Just a few things to keep in mind when it comes to your unlimited veggie allotment:

➤ Don't forget that I identify some vegetables as Angel Carbs. Corn, beans, peas and chickpeas are in this category and so must be limited to four to seven weekly.

➤ Also, there are certain vegetables that are too pickable, poppable, unstoppable to consider in the unlimited category. That would include cherry tomatoes and baby carrots. I've had clients eat massive quantities of both these veggies, which is not only, believe it or not, too many calories but also a reinforcement of bad eating behavior. Of course you can enjoy cherry tomatoes and baby carrots. But only in small handful amounts or in salads. That's it. No big bowls on the counter to be picked at each time you pass by, all day long.

➤ The best veggies to snack on are celery, cucumbers and raw peppers. Why? Because they have less sugar than some other veggies (like carrots) and because they require some prep, they are not pickable or poppable.

➤ Crudités at parties can be trigger foods because they can become pickable, poppable and there's usually dip nearby. It's obviously better than cheese, but if you know that the baby carrots are going to lead to the onion dip, then steer clear.

➤ If you're cooking veggies at home, steam them; if you're ordering them in a restaurant, if they don't offer steamed, sautéed is fine. But avoid veggies that are creamed or fried.

➤ You can have unlimited veggies daily.

PROTEIN Protein, in moderation, is prime diet food. It keeps you satisfied. It takes longer to digest than carbs—about four hours versus only about two for carbs—so it helps keep you fuller, longer. In fact a very recent study found that people who ate protein for breakfast lost more weight and kept it off compared with people who ate carbs, even though the calorie intake in both groups' breakfasts was the same. Protein—the lean protein sources that I recommend—also tends to be binge proof. You'll find lean protein in fish, turkey, chicken, egg whites, nonfat yogurt and lean beef.

Soups!

How do you handle soups?

Soups can be a great addition to your diet if you choose wisely. Clear, light soups can make a good appetizer choice because they help to fill you up. Other types of soups are still good choices, but the ingredients will determine how you count them in your daily diet. Check the Angel Carb list in the Blueprint. If the soup contains anything from the Familiar Angel Carbs—brown rice, couscous, grains, potato, wheat noodles, etc.—it counts as an Angel Carb. I would skip a soup-and-sandwich combo at lunch to avoid having a double carb meal. Rather, choose a salad to accompany the soup. And of course steer clear of creamy soups and salty soups.

Include some protein in every meal. In addition to protein at breakfast promoting weight loss, I've found that people who tend to eat only carbs for breakfast can struggle with mood swings and hunger. Eating protein at *every* meal, not only breakfast, helps keep you on an even keel, stabilizes your blood sugar and prevents mood swings.

Again, as I mentioned above, vegetarian protein choices include all beans, as well as tofu and meat substitutes. So here are the guidelines on protein:

➤ Pick protein that's grilled, steamed, broiled, baked or poached. Avoid fried or breaded protein.

➤ Choose low- or nonfat Greek yogurt when available because it's higher in protein and has far less sugar than regular yogurt.

➤ Avoid nuts or nut butters except for individual serving packets like Justin's peanut butter (see pages 286–287).

➤ Buy individual ¼ pound bags of turkey (fresh or low-sodium is best). They'll come in handy for a quick lunch and also for a nighttime go-to snack. I order two or three individual bags at the deli counter regularly.

➤ Avoid cheese! You know why. A little weeny piece of cheese can have 100 calories. And you can't stop eating it, right? It's OK to have a few shaves of Parmesan or pecorino on your salad, or the snack cheeses I recommend in the shopping list, but stay away from big bricks of cheddar or that baked brie they pass at parties.

➤ Remember portion sizes for protein are approximately the size of a cell phone. Women should have one protein serving at lunch and one at dinner. Men can double this amount. If you have a lot of weight to lose you don't need to stick to the smaller volume of protein the first few weeks because you will be too hungry. If you're a veteran dieter with less than twenty pounds to lose, stick with the lower protein portion. Breakfast protein would be 4–6 egg whites, 2–3 whole eggs or ½ to 1 cup of yogurt.

➤ You should have protein at each meal.

BEVERAGES   Here's what you need to know about beverages in three words: Drink more water! Skip the juice and cut down on the coffee. Reduce caffeine in the afternoon by enjoying herbal teas. And drink, drink, drink your water. Water makes a big difference in weight loss. I've seen it time and again with clients. People who ate relatively well but never touched a drop of water found that once they followed my water intake guidelines, they began to shed pounds. Researchers aren't sure why water intake can boost weight loss. Is it the fact that water can help fill you up so you eat less? Or does water have an effect on your metabolism such that it stimulates calorie burning? Whatever, it definitely works.

I instruct clients to have 2 liters of water daily. You should try to consume that first liter before lunch. I call it "LBL": liter by lunch. Get in your second liter by the end of the day. No other liquids—seltzer, tea, etc.,—count toward your water goal. It's water, water, water.

At the same time that you're increasing water, you should also try to limit caffeine. Coffee or tea in the morning or right after lunch is fine. But caffeine in the late afternoon can have an effect on your sleep patterns and we now know that people who sleep fewer than seven to nine hours at night have difficulty losing weight. Caffeine can also make you crave food—usually sweets or carbs—when the rush of energy wears off.

Finally, avoid diet sodas. The final verdict still isn't in, but

Two Water Tips

Sippy Bottle: I might mention that drinking an ample amount of water doesn't come naturally to me. For one thing, I hate drinking water from a glass. I know this is odd, but in fact some of my clients feel the same way. Here's a tip that makes all the difference to me and maybe it will work for you. I use what I think of as an adult "sippy cup": a Nalgene BPA-free water bottle. It comes in 24- and 32-ounce sizes, and I love them because they have these little pop-up straws. Of course you can find other, comparable, brands. I fill mine first thing in the morning and start sipping before I even have my coffee. I save on bottled water, do something for the environment and satisfy my wicked oral fixation. My water bottle has saved me millions of calories. Of course, if you are comfortable drinking from a glass or anything else, go for it! Ice water? Room temp? It doesn't make a difference as far as weight loss is concerned. Just make sure to get your total ounces in daily.

Boxed Water: If you prefer to drink water from a plastic bottle but keep forgetting to pick one up, consider ordering a case of water for your home or office. You'd be surprised how helpful it can be to have those 1.5 liter bottles at home or at work. I know that it's not the most earth-friendly solution (for that I highly recommend your own Nalgene bottle), but for many people a fresh bottle of water at hand makes the difference between great hydration and none. If it's going to help you hydrate and lose weight, then go for it!

they seem to have negative effects on overall health as well as on weight loss. I tell clients if you're desperate for a diet soda, wait until you've had your 64 ounces of water. (Usually by then they've lost interest.)

➤ Drink 64 ounces of water daily. Avoid juice and soda; limit caffeinated beverages and diet soda.

ALCOHOL   When I first began working with people who were trying to lose weight, I usually made the traditional recommendation: Give up alcohol. After all, alcohol has calories and little nutritional benefits. It's our favorite source of "empty calories." But for most of my clients, this recommendation turned out to be a deal breaker. So I had to figure out a way to help them lose weight even though they were going to insist on their wine with dinner or cocktail before. Here's what I came up with and it works: One drink is free. You can have one drink a day without it counting. By drink, I mean a nonsweetened alcoholic drink like wine, light beer, vodka or scotch. Avoid the margaritas, pina coladas or cosmos and their like. They're all full of sugar and calories. After that first free drink, any additional drink counts as a Carb. You can have a second drink, but you have to count it in your daily tally. Keep in mind that if alcohol affects your eating behavior, you have to be sensible about how much you drink. If you find that two drinks melts your inhibitions and you lose control of what you eat, then obviously you have to restrain yourself if you really want to lose weight. Some people have the opposite response: Alcohol makes them lose their appetite. This still doesn't mean you can drink too much because overindulgence can prompt a Plunge the next day. Hangovers give you more than a headache: You can find yourself irresistibly drawn to carbs the day after and it can be a struggle to get back on track. I have some more particular tips about alcohol in the Dine-Out Devils on page 220.

> Your first drink is free; any after that counts
>   as a carb.

FATS AND OILS   Fats and oils count. But your focus on this category will depend on how much weight you have to lose. If you have twenty to thirty pounds or more to lose, then don't get hung up too much on fats and oils. Of course you should avoid all fried food and creamed sauces and anything that you know has lots of fat in it.

Most of my clients who only have five to ten pounds to lose are already conscious of fats in their diet, and most are doing a fairly good job of avoiding creamy and fried foods as well as fatty meats. To fine-tune your calorie intake you'll need to focus just a bit more on fats and oils, particularly the dressings. You'll be eating a lot more salads and vegetables and therefore a lot more dressings. Some dressings pack a whopping amount of calories. So take a look at the dressings in your fridge and make sure they are "lite" or low fat (see page 284 for specific brand suggestions). I always recommend choosing oil and vinegar, and going very light on the oil, when you're a guest or in another situation where the choice is only creamy or "mystery" dressing. Remember too that you don't need to drown your salad in dressing. A serving of salad dressing is actually two tablespoons and many of us glug, glug, glug on much more than that. Try using just a drizzle of dressing and mix it well and you might find that you can cut your dressing intake in half without any loss of flavor. It's helpful to measure out dressing by the tablespoon until you can judge an appropriate serving size.

A note on olive oil: Many of my clients have read that olive oil, as part of a Mediterranean diet, is good for you. Well, yes, that's true. But dipping a loaf of bread into a quarter cup of olive oil is not exactly a healthy move (or a Mediterranean diet, for that matter!). In fact, my husband and I always used to toss our veggies into some olive oil before roasting. One day we measured how much oil we were using on the veggies for just the two of us and it added up to 6 tablespoons! That's 720 calories! While olive oil may well be healthier for your heart than a margarine that contains trans fat, it's still a fat, so use it sparingly. One trick I often use at home is to buy a healthy "lite" or low-fat dressing and then decant it and mix in additional vinegar, either balsamic or sherry or whatever vinegar seems to suit the dressing. This reduces the calories but still punches up the flavor of greens.

While we're on the subject of salads, I should mention that although salads are an excellent choice, they could also be very high in calories if you aren't careful with your ingredients. A Cobb salad, for example, can pack up to 1,200 calories by the time you add the egg and bacon and cheese. If you're going to enjoy a Cobb salad, or any salad with fats and proteins mixed in, my recommendation is to limit yourself to two fats: So in a Cobb salad you might have the avocado and dressing and skip the cheese, bacon and egg yolk. Check out my salad bar recipes on page 242 for some great, tasty, low-cal salad suggestions.

It's not only with our salads that we encounter fats and oils. There are also all the fried foods, creamy sauces and pastas with oils, but it's pretty obvious that you should avoid these foods if you want to lose weight.

➤ Avoid fatty foods. Choose lower-fat salad dressings and use them sparingly.

CONDIMENTS Oh, please . . . what's so bad about a smidge of ketchup? Or a light schmear of mayo? Well, the bad news is that just a tablespoon of mayo has 100 calories and 10 grams of fat! Of course if you stopped at one tablespoon it might be acceptable, but have you ever watched how much mayo they can put on a sandwich at the deli? Here's one way to think of it: three tablespoons of mayo is 300 calories and that's close to a Whopper Jr. at 360 calories! Some sandwiches have virtual boatloads of mayo. So I've made a "pick" and a "skip" list of condiments on the Blueprint Chart, and this is a little area where you can save big calories. So, for example, mustard (low cal, some health benefits) is a "pick"; barbeque sauce (high in calories and sugar) is a "skip."

Does this mean you can never again have anything with barbeque sauce on it? No, of course not. But it does mean that you have to manage your condiment intake. The easiest way to do this is to count a significant condiment intake as an Angel Carb. So if you are the kind of person who every once in a blue moon indulges in french fries that are just swimming in ketchup, well, that ketchup counts as an Angel Carb. (The fries are total Devils.)

➤ Use sparingly.

SNACKS Snacks are the clever tools you can rely on to save you from the various Devils. A properly timed snack can be a real lifeline. I find it useful to have a specific category designated as "snack" just to distinguish snacks from the other food categories. I don't want you to get too hung up on "Is it a fiber? A fruit?" Don't worry about it. It's just a snack.

Snacks are under 200 calories. They are typically finite foods—in portion-controlled amounts, like energy bars. A few good snack choices include a Gnu bar, a Larabar, a Luna bar, a Nature Valley granola bar, or a 1.3-ounce bag of Glenny's Soy Crisps, two fiber crackers and two Laughing Cow light cheeses or just a hand fruit. (For a complete list of snacks, see page 286.)

Not everyone needs a snack. Some people do just fine on their three meals. Others really need something in the afternoon to get them over the hunger hump. Many people snack mindlessly and, in fact, this is why they come to see me in the first place. Your food journal will help you figure out if a snack will help you because it will show you the times of day when you tend to overeat. In addition to reviewing your food journal, you can take my snack test: When you eat an afternoon snack, does it help you eat less at dinner? If yes, the snack is a good strategy for you; if no, you should probably skip the snack and stick to three meals.

When you're picking a snack, consider what you're currently eating: If a cookie is your current snack of choice, you should upgrade to a bar. If you're already eating a bar, try switching up to a hand fruit. The idea is to bump up the quality and bump down the calories in your current snack. An apple, at 60 calories and lots of fiber, is usually a better choice than a bar. But a bar can be convenient and satisfying.

Don't forget that you can Phase Eat snacks. If it's easier for you to stick to just one snack option for weeks on end, that's fine. If you prefer to vary your snacks, that's fine too.

One more tip on snacks: they're not only for the afternoon. A snack can be an extremely useful tool to help you stick to your guns when you're facing a big business dinner, a cocktail party, a buffet, a gala event . . . any situation that involves lots of food that's going to be difficult to resist. Prepare yourself in advance for these events by enjoying a snack and a good portion of water thirty to forty-five minutes before you head to your event. You'll be surprised by how much this helps.

By the way, for those of you who have blood sugar issues and must eat every two or three hours, you should add in a mid-morning snack. The key is to keep them under 80 calories. A small piece of fruit, string cheese, ten almonds, one Mini Babybel or Laughing Cow cheese with one GG cracker are all good choices.

Creative afternoon snack options under 200 calories (pick only one). There are many more options in the shopping list:

✓ Mix an 80-calorie 0% fat Greek yogurt with 1 T of organic spinach powder dip and eat with a cut-up cucumber.

✓ Take a 100-calorie bag of popcorn and add Tabasco or 1 Mini Babybel cheese.

✓ Try Matt's Munchies individually wrapped snacks. They take some time to peel, but some have as few as 90 calories.

✓ Have an Annie Chun's roasted seaweed snack, wasabi style; it has just 60 calories and is a good choice to eat during kids' dinner before your "adult" dinner.

✓ Have an apple with a 100-calorie pack Justin's nut butter.

✓ Eat a Sabra or Tribe 100-calorie pack hummus with cut-up veggies.

✓ Heat up a 100-calorie microwavable bag of Dora the Explorer edamame.

✓ Take a 100-calorie bag of raw almonds and toast them.

✓ Eat two celery stalks with two Laughing Cow light cheeses (try the flavored ones to spice things up a bit—blue cheese is great with the celery).

I Love, Love, Love Gnu Bars!

They are great snacks: One bar has between 130 and 140 calories, depending on flavor, and it gives you *half* your daily fiber. It can also double as a breakfast bar that, with a piece of fruit, makes a good on-the-go breakfast. Some of my clients have joined the "Joy of Fiber Club" on the Gnu Web site, which gives you a discount on the purchase as well as free shipping. If you find a food that you like, it always makes sense to keep a good supply on hand to make your life and your diet easier. See www .gnufoods.com.

➤ In general, you can have one afternoon snack—usually under 200 calories—daily.

Frozen Dinners

You'll notice that I include frozen dinners as Angel Carbs in the Blueprint. Frozen dinners are what I call finite foods—foods that come in limited portion sizes. They are a dieter's best friend. Frozen dinners are perhaps the gold-star finite foods. Frozen entrées can rescue you when you're too tired to cook, when you get home late with nothing to eat in the house or when you simply need an easy, portion-controlled meal to help you stay on track. You can also pop in a frozen dinner on a weekend when you're in the mood for something more interesting for lunch than a simple sandwich. Frozen entrées can also be a great choice for those times when you're just craving a pasta meal but don't want to take the risk of overeating—something too easy to do with carryout pasta or a homemade pasta dinner. And at my house, frozen dinners help me out when my steak-loving hungry husband wants a big chunk of cow and I don't.

Here is another benefit of frozen dinners: They reeducate you about portion sizes. We get so used to our giant servings in restaurants and at home that we've begun to think they're normal. They're not! Serving sizes in many restaurants are enough to serve two or more. Take a look at the protein in a typical frozen dinner that features chicken or fish: You'll see that the size of the protein serving is about the size of a cell phone. This is an appropriate serving size. Keep this in mind when you're cooking at home. Would the meal you're about to dig into fit in a frozen dinner tray?

Frozen dinners also help reintroduce people to healthy carbs. So many clients who come to me are carb-phobic. They are overweight and only eat protein-and-veggie diets. When I suggest they try a 300-calorie frozen pasta dinner (400 for a male), they're shocked. But when they do it, they lose weight. Why? It's lower in volume than they're used to eating, even though it's totally satisfying. It's also lower in calories than the order of steamed chicken and broccoli in brown sauce that they might be getting from their local Chinese place.

Choose frozen entrées that are no more than 300 calories if you're a woman and no more than 400 if you're a man. I'm a big fan of Amy's organic frozen entrées because they're really tasty and, of course, they're organic. But there are other brands that are also delicious and easy to find in any supermarket. If you are a male or have more than twenty pounds to lose and find that a frozen entrée doesn't fill you up, you can add a green salad or some frozen veggies and call it a meal.

And, by the way, many clients worry about the amount of sodium in frozen meals. While it's true that many frozen meals are too high in sodium, the ones I recommend are not. I'm careful to choose meals that are at the low end of the sodium range so you can be confident that they're healthy. I might also mention that if you're following the Blueprint, your daily sodium intake is probably far below that of a typical American.

Below is a list of the brands of frozen entrées my clients and

I agree are the most flavorful, healthy and satisfying. A tip: I've discovered that most of these brands taste best when baked in a toaster oven. This reduces cooking time over a conventional oven (also seems less wasteful than turning on the big oven) but will take longer than in a microwave. They're especially good for lunch, for a light dinner after a cocktail party or after you've had a big lunch. (Check page 285 for many other suggestions.)

KASHI: Black Bean Mango, Lime Cilantro Shrimp, Sweet & Sour Chicken

AMY'S: Light & Lean Pasta & Veggies, Light & Lean Soft Taco Fiesta, Vegetable Lasagne, Mexican Tamale Pie, Spinach Feta in a Pocket Sandwich, Stuffed Pasta Shells

ORGANIC BISTRO: Wild Alaskan Salmon, Ginger Chicken, Sesame Ginger Wild Salmon Bowl

TRADER JOE'S: Reduced Guilt Tilapia with Fava Beans, Reduced Guilt Mac & Cheese, Grilled Eggplant Parmesan, Chicken Tikka Masala

FRENCH MEADOW: Orange Mango Chicken, Garlic Chicken, Fragrant Curry Chicken

Two low-calorie choices are especially good for lunch or post-party or as a late-night dinner:

Amy's Mexican Tamale Pie (150 calories)

Moo Moo's Vegetable Lasagna (170 calories)

Sample Menus

Here are sample three-week menus that offer suggestions for what you can eat on the diet. When I drew up the menus, I tried to make them as close as possible to the typical menus of my clients.[2] The menu plans for females emphasize small portion sizes, lower-fat options, more veggie and fish options, brown-bag lunches and more frozen options. The menus for males are higher in calories and have bigger meals, more dining-out options, more red meat options and higher-calorie energy bars.

You'll see that in the first two weeks of the menus I've emphasized Phase Eating with just two or three options for breakfast and a limited number of lunch options. Then in the third week I roll out alternative ideas. So if you don't see choices that appeal to you in the first two weeks, make sure you check out the final week. For dinner, see what appeals to you in terms of your tastes and your lifestyle. If you're out every night, you can concentrate on the chapter "Dine-Out Devil" for good restaurant choices. If you're eating at home, you can check out my recipes and frozen choices.

The Basic Formula for Each Meal:

BREAKFAST: Fiber + protein + fruit

LUNCH: Protein + veggies + optional carb + optional fruit

AFTERNOON SNACK: Bar or fruit

DINNER: Protein + veggie + optional carb

FINAL SNACK: 1 fruit only within 20 minutes of dinner, then kitchen closed!

2 Although I of course considered calories while drawing up the menu plans, I don't encourage readers to count calories. As a very general rule, females do best with a weight loss plan that's close to 1,200 calories and males do best with a plan that's close to 1,800 calories daily. Obviously this can vary greatly depending on current weight, metabolism and energy expenditure.

Female Three-Week Sample Menus

	Monday	Tuesday	Wednesday	Thursday
Breakfast	2 hard-boiled eggs, 2GG crackers, 1 apple	6 oz 0% Greek yogurt with ¼ cup Kashi Go Lean and ½ cup blueberries	2 hard-boiled eggs, 2GG crackers, 1 apple	6 oz 0% Greek yogurt with ¼ cup Kashi Go Lean and ½ cup blueberries
Lunch	*From deli:* 4 oz sliced turkey sandwich on 2 slices whole wheat bread with raw veggies (lettuce/tomato/cucumbers/sprouts) and mustard	*Build a salad from a salad bar:* Lettuce, nonstarchy raw veggies, 3 oz lean protein (grilled chicken, turkey, egg whites, tofu, salmon, shrimp, dry tuna) with balsamic vinegar and 1 T olive oil* 2GG crackers	*Starbucks:* Farmers market salad (add 2GG crackers) plus unsweetened tea	*Build a salad from a salad bar:* Lettuce, nonstarchy raw veggies, 3 oz lean protein (grilled chicken, turkey, egg whites, tofu, salmon, shrimp, dry tuna) with balsamic vinegar and 1 T olive oil* 2GG crackers
Snack	Gnu bar	1 fruit	Gnu bar	1 fruit
Dinner	*Pick up dinner at market:* ¼ rotisserie chicken (no skin), one small side of steamed or roasted veggies (nonstarchy, not soaked in oil) Small side green salad with 1 T olive oil and balsamic vinegar OR 1 orange	*Out for dinner:* 1 glass of wine Arugula salad (2 cups) with 1 oz shaved parmesan with 2 T balsamic vinaigrette (ask for light on the dressing) 4-6 oz grilled branzino with sautéed spinach (dish came in a sauce) Optional: 2 spoonfuls of shared vegetables Berries for dessert	*Frozen meal:* Amy's Light 'n Lean black bean and cheese enchilada 1 orange	*Veggie Night:* Large baked sweet potato plus 2 cups of steamed broccoli and cauliflower 1 baked apple with cinnamon

*Appropriate salad dressings include balsamic vinegar+1 T olive oil, rice vinegar+1 T olive oil, 1 T olive oil+lemon juice, 1–2 T of any light balsamic dressing of choice (Newman's, Annie's)

Friday	Saturday	Sunday
2 hard-boiled eggs, 2GG crackers, 1 apple	6 oz 0% Greek yogurt with ¼ cup Kashi Go Lean mixed in plus ¼ cup pomegranate seeds	Optional: 1 serving fruit OR your choice of breakfast bar**
Brown-bag lunch: Homemade low-fat tuna salad using 1 T low-fat mayo and 4 oz of chunk light tuna in water on whole wheat La Tortilla wrap with raw veggies (lettuce/ tomato/ cucumbers/ sprouts)*	*California Pizza Kitchen:* Half the roasted veggie salad with shrimp	*Out to Brunch:* Egg white vegetable omelet with 1 slice American cheese, sliced tomatoes 1 optional piece of Canadian bacon Small fruit salad
Gnu bar	Tall skim latte and 1 fruit	Optional: 100-calorie pack of almonds plus 1 fruit
Cook dinner at home: Chicken Parm Lite (see recipe) 4 oz chicken baked with spinach and shirataki noodles Salmon stir fry 1 glass wine 1 cup berries	*Out for dinner:* 2 glasses of wine Beet and goat cheese salad with 1 oz goat cheese 5 oz grilled halibut with asparagus in sauce and shared side of sautéed mushrooms	*Ordering in Chinese food:* 4 oz steamed moo shoo chicken with lettuce wraps and 1 T Hoisin sauce or low sodium soy sauce Use 1 La Tortilla wrap instead for one of the wraps 1 orange

*For sandwiches made at home use Thomas's Light, high-fiber, whole-grain English muffins (100 calories each), La Tortilla Factory whole wheat wraps, any other whole wheat bread where 2 slices are 100 calories or less (when out opt for wheat/rye bread, skip wraps)

**Recommended breakfast bars: Cascadian Farms Almond Butter, Gnu, Oskri Fiber Bar, Organic Fiber Bar

Female Three-Week Sample Menus

	Monday: PROTEIN RECOVERY DAY*	Tuesday	Wednesday	Thursday
Breakfast	2 hard-boiled eggs or 6 egg white mushroom omelet (no cheese)	1 packet oatmeal (100 calories) with water with cinnamon and 1 small diced apple cooked in** Optional: plus 1 T ground flaxseed	½ cup 2% Break-stone's mini cottage cheese 2 GG 1 fruit	Starbucks: Perfect oatmeal Iced Americano/ skim milk Optional fruit
Lunch	3 oz sliced turkey or chicken over mixed green salad with cucumbers, mushrooms, balsamic vinegar plus 1 T olive oil	Brown-bag lunch: 4 oz sliced turkey on light wheat bread with raw veggies (lettuce/ tomato/ cucumbers/ sprouts), 1 slice of low-fat cheese and mustard 1 apple	Medium (12 oz) chicken vegetable soup (or any low-fat, dairy-free, low-sodium soup) 2 GG crackers and optional fruit	Out for lunch: Tuna Nicoise salad (no potato) with 3–4 oz tuna, oil/vinegar dressing
Snack	1 orange or small grapefruit or ¼ lb sliced turkey	1 Matt's Munchies fruit leather	Kind bar	1 fruit + 1 Babybel light cheese
Dinner	Out for dinner: Mixed green salad with 2 T dressing 4–6 oz grilled fish/chicken or steak with steamed spinach or asparagus	Frozen dinner: Organic Bistro wild salmon Fruit for dessert	Ordering in from Italian restaurant (at the office or home): Some of a shared mixed green salad with light vinaigrette Shrimp marinara (6 large shrimp, ½ cup marinara sauce, no pasta), can top with crushed red pepper flakes 1 cup of sautéed broccoli rabe	Quick prep dinner: 1 veggie burger plus Arnold 100 cal sandwich thin, 2 sides steamed veggies 1 orange

*Recovery Days are described on page 73. They are not mandatory; this is just an example of how one would work in real life.

**Can be substituted for any 1 serving of fruit—for instance: ¾ cup raspberries, 1 cup strawberries, ½ banana, 1 small apple cut into chunks and cooked in oatmeal, or 1 medium orange on the side

Friday	Saturday	Sunday
½ cup 2% Breakstone's mini cottage cheese 2 GG 1 fruit	Breakfast on the go: Gnu bar Optional fruit	Optional: 1 fruit OR your choice of breakfast bar*
Le Pain Quotidien: 6-vegetable garden gluten-free quiche	*Frozen lunch:* Amy's Mexican Tamale pie Optional raw veggies cut up	*Out for brunch:* Eggs Benedict—skip the sauce and the English muffin (share fruit salad w/ table)
2% blueberry Greek yogurt	100-calorie pack of almonds Hungry before dinner: 2GG crackers and 1 Laughing Cow light cheese	Tall skim latte 1 cup of cut up red peppers 100-calorie mini bag of light popcorn with 1 Babybel light cheese
Pizza night: 1 slice of a 12-inch thin crust cheese pizza Mixed green salad w/ balsamic vinaigrette and 1 cup of steamed veggies if still hungry 1 glass of wine 17 frozen grapes	*Out for sushi dinner:* 2 glasses of wine Green salad (light on the dressing, use ½ dressing) or miso soup Optional: Oshitashi 4 pieces sashimi and 1 salmon/tuna/yellowtail etc. roll (nonfried, nonspicy) Shared sorbet with table	*Cooking at home:* Super Scallops (see recipe page 273)—served with mixed greens, steamed aspara-gus and ½ cup brown rice 1 glass of wine 1 orange

*Recommended breakfast bars: Cascadian Farms Almond Butter, Gnu, Oskri Fiber Bar, Organic Fiber Bar

Female Three-Week Sample Menus

	Monday: VOLUME- CONTROLLED RECOVERY DAY	Tuesday	Wednesday	Thursday
Breakfast	0% Greek yogurt with ½ cup Kashi Go Lean and ½ cup berries	*Breakfast on-the-go:* Gnu Bar and apple Extra dry tall skim cappuccino	*Homemade smoothie:* 6 oz plain or 0% Greek yogurt, ice, 1 T ground flaxseed, 1 cup frozen berries, 1 t natural peanut butter	½ cup 2% Breakstone's mini cottage cheese 2 GG crackers 1 fruit
Lunch	*From deli:* 4 oz sliced turkey sandwich on 2 slices whole wheat bread with raw veggies (lettuce/tomato/cucumbers/sprouts) and mustard Piece of fruit	*Cosi:* Bombay chicken salad, request that it is "light-ened up," add in 2 GG crackers Optional fruit	*Brown-bag lunch:* Leftover chicken (3 oz) and sautéed veggies from last night's dinner + ½ cup black beans over mixed salad greens with balsamic vinegar + 1 T olive oil*	*Out for lunch:* Endive salad Tuna tartare appetizer Side of steamed asparagus
Snack	Gnu bar	100-calorie bag raw almonds and an apple	Kind bar	1 Matt's Munchies
Dinner	*Frozen dinner:* Trader Joe's baked eggplant parm 1 cup berries	*Mexican dinner out:* 2 T guacamole with sliced jicama (no chips) 4 oz chicken or shrimp fajita, no tortilla, no rice, sautéed onions and peppers and ½ cup black beans 1 vodka soda with lime	*Pick up from market:* 4 oz poached salmon 1 cup brussels sprouts ½ cup quinoa salad 1 orange sliced with cinnamon	*Frozen dinner:* Amy's low-sodium brown rice and veggie bowl 1 baked apple with cinnamon

*Recovery Days are described on page 73. They are not mandatory; this is just an example of how one would work in real life.

Friday	Saturday	Sunday
2 FiberRich crackers with 100-calorie packet of Justin's nut butter and sliced ½ banana	Making pancakes for the kids: Oatmeal pancakes (see recipe page 272) OR 2 Vans Lite waffles with ½ cup 1% whipped cottage cheese plus ½ cup blueberries	Making eggs at home for brunch: Homemade 6 egg white omelet (made with Pam) with 1–2 cups of spinach and onions and 1 oz soy cheddar cheese 2 GG crackers
Chopped green salad with lean protein: lettuce, nonstarchy raw veggies, 3 oz lean protein (grilled chicken, turkey, egg whites, tofu, salmon, shrimp, dry tuna) with balsamic vinegar and 1 T olive oil* 2 GG crackers	*Subway lunch:* Subway 6-inch wheat roll (ask for it to be "scooped out") with sliced turkey or chicken, lettuce, tomato, mustard and one slice cheese 1 pack of apple slices	
2 GG crackers and 1 Cabot light cheese wheel	Kopali Organics Superfoods mix	100-calorie container of hummus with 2 FiberRich crackers and raw veggies Later snack: 1 fruit
Steakhouse dinner: 2 glasses wine Tomato and red onion salad (with 2 T vinaigrette or balsamic vinegar) Order smallest size lean steak, usually 8 oz, but aim to eat 4–6 oz (share/save the rest) Shared vegetable sides: sautéed mushrooms and steamed broccoli	*Ordering in Thai:* 1 cup tom yum soup 1 piece of chicken satay Green papaya salad with chicken or shrimp (carb in sauce/dressing) (No rice)	*Cooking at home:* Angel Chicken Paillard (see recipe page 274): chicken prepared with panko and unprocessed bran served with salad Sautéd mushrooms on the side 17 frozen grapes

*Appropriate salad dressings include: balsamic vinegar+1 TBST olive oil, rice vinegar+1 TBST olive oil, 1 TBSP olive oil+lemon juice, 1-2 T of any light balsamic dressing of choice (Newman's, Annie's)

Male Three-Week Sample Menus

	Monday	**Tuesday**	**Wednesday**	**Thursday**
Breakfast	6 egg whites with 1 slice cheese, 2 FiberRich crackers, plus apple	1 cup 2% Greek yogurt with ½ cup Kashi Go Lean and 1 sliced banana**	6 egg whites with 1 slice cheese, 2 FiberRich crackers, plus apple	**Starbucks:** Grande skim latte, Gnu bar and fruit
Lunch	*From deli:* Sliced turkey sandwich on 2 slices whole wheat bread with raw veggies (lettuce/tomato/cucumbers/sprouts) and mustard, and 1 slice of cheese or avocado*	*Chopped salad bar:* mixed greens, 3 nonstarchy raw veggies, lean protein double order (grilled chicken, turkey, egg whites, tofu, salmon, shrimp, dry tuna) with light balsamic vinaigrette 2 Fiber Rich crackers	*Le Pain Quotidien:* Grilled chicken cobb salad w/out the cheese and ½ dressing plus unsweetened iced tea	Greek salad, no grape leaves, light on feta with grilled chicken, light red-wine vinaigrette dressing
Snack	Kashi Go Lean Roll Bar	1 fruit	Luna protein bar	1 fruit
Dinner	*Pick up dinner at market:* ¼–½ rotisserie chicken (no skin), 1 cup of steamed or roasted veggies (non-starchy, not soaked in oil) and small green salad	*Out for dinner:* 2 glasses wine Appetizer tuna tartare Grilled veal chop with sautéed broccoli rabe Shared fruit plate for dessert	*Frozen meal:* French Meadow chicken curry with 2 cups of steamed vegetables and small green salad with 1T olive oil and balsamic vinegar* 1 cup berries	*Quick prep dinner:* Applegate Farms frozen turkey burger patty with 1 slice 1% cheese on Arnold sandwich thin plus 2 cups of steamed vegetables and small side green salad with 1 T olive oil and balsamic vinegar 1 light beer 1 orange

*For sandwiches you can use: Thomas's Light, high-fiber, whole-grain English muffins (100 cal each), La Tortilla Factory whole-wheat wraps, any other bread whole wheat bread where 2 slices are 100 calories or less (see shopping list for alternatives)

**Can be substituted for any 1 serving of fruit—for instance: ¾ cup raspberries, 1 cup strawberries, ½ banana, 1 small apple cut into chunks and cooked in oatmeal, or 1 medium orange on the side

Friday	Saturday	Sunday
1 cup 2% Greek yogurt with ½ cup Kashi Go Lean and 1 banana sliced*	2 scrambled eggs with salsa, 1 T 1% shredded cheese, 1 T black bean dip, 1 La Tortilla Factory wrap	Optional: 1 serving fruit OR your choice of breakfast bar**
Starbucks: Turkey and swiss sandwich (390 cals) plus apple and unsweetened iced tea	*California Pizza Kitchen:* Full Caesar with grilled chicken and substitute dressing for the fat-free vinaigrette	*Out to brunch:* Omelet with goat cheese, mushrooms, spinach 1–2 pieces of Canadian bacon Optional: Fruit salad
Mojo bar	Glenny's Soy Crisps with 1 fruit plus 2 FiberRich crackers with 1 Laughing Cow light cheese	100-calorie pack of almonds plus 1 fruit (optional)
Cook dinner at home: Mustard-crusted steak (page 277) (8 oz) Small green salad (2 cups lettuce with 1 T olive oil and balsamic vinegar) Steamed asparagus 2 glasses red wine 1 cup berries	*Out for dinner:* Vodka on the rocks Grilled octopus appetizer Sesame-crusted seared tuna with sautéed bok choy Optional: 2–3 spoonfuls of shared side vegetables and fruit plate for dessert	*Ordering in Chinese food:* Bowl of hot-and-sour or egg-drop soup (12 oz) Steamed chicken (8 oz) moo shoo with lettuce wraps and 1 T Hoisin sauce or low-sodium soy sauce 1–2 spare ribs (sauce) 1 orange

*Recommended breakfast bars: Cascadian Farms Almond Butter, Gnu, Oskri Fiber Bar, Organic Fiber Bar

**Can be substituted for any 1 serving of fruit—for instance: ¾ cup raspberries, 1 cup strawberries, ½ banana, 1 small apple cut into chunks and cooked in oatmeal, or 1 medium orange on the side

Male Three-Week Sample Menus

	Monday: PROTEIN RECOVERY DAY*	Tuesday	Wednesday	Thursday
Breakfast	3 scrambled eggs or 6 egg white mushroom omelet (no cheese)	1 cup plain oatmeal cooked with water or ½ cup of skim or almond milk, 1 cup berries plus 1 T ground flaxseed (optional)	1 cup 1% cottage cheese and 2 FiberRich crackers 1 fruit	*Starbucks:* Perfect oatmeal with nuts (240 calories) plus apple
Lunch	6 oz turkey or chicken plus 2 egg whites over 3 cups mixed green salad with cucumbers, mushrooms, 1 T olive oil and balsamic vinegar	*Sushi lunch:* 1 salmon naruto roll (sashimi wrapped in cucumber, no rice), 1 yellowtail scallion hand roll with cucumber instead of rice, 1 small green salad with 2 T dressing	Medium size (12 oz) turkey or vegetable chili or lentil soup with side of small green salad or sautéed vegetables (1 cup)	*Out for lunch:* Rocket salad appetizer Grilled branzino with sautéed asparagus on the side Espresso
Snack	1 orange or 1 small grapefruit ¼ lb sliced turkey	100-calorie pack of almonds 1 fruit	Balance bar	1 fruit plus 2 Babybel light cheeses
Dinner	*Out for dinner:* Small mixed green salad with light oil and vinegar dressing 8–10 oz lean grilled steak (filet or sirloin) served over 1 cup steamed spinach	*Ordering in from Italian restaurant (at the office or home):* Small mixed green salad with light oil and vinegar dressing Shrimp marinara (6 large shrimp, ½ cup marinara sauce, no pasta), can top with crushed red pepper flakes 1 piece of chicken cacciatore 1 cup of sautéed broccoli rabe	*Frozen dinner:* Kashi sweet & sour chicken plus 2 cups of steamed vegetables Small side green salad with 1 T olive oil and balsamic vinegar 1 orange	*Out for dinner at a tapas restaurant:* 2 glasses of wine Share lean protein or vegetable tapas—all the sauce in the food counts as 1 carb

*Can be substituted for any 1 serving of fruit—for instance: ¾ cup raspberries, 1 cup strawberries, ½ banana, 1 small apple cut into chunks and cooked in oatmeal, or 1 medium orange on the side

Friday	Saturday	Sunday
1 cup 1% cottage cheese and 2 FiberRich crackers 1 fruit	Light wheat English muffin, 2T peanut butter with ½ banana OR Amy's breakfast burrito (6 oz.) plus one fruit of choice	Optional: 1 fruit OR your choice of breakfast bar
Out for lunch: Mixed green salad with raw veggies and 2 T balsamic vinaigrette Hamburger (no bun, no cheese) with tomato, lettuce, onion	*On the road fast food:* McDonald's grilled chicken Caesar salad with Newman's light vinaigrette dressing instead of Caesar dressing (1 packet)	*Out for brunch:* Eggs Benedict, skip the sauce, only eat ½ the English muffin
Kashi Crunchy bar Apple closer to dinner	1.3 oz bag Glenny's Soy Crisps Hungry before dinner: 2 slices of turkey plus 2 FiberRich crackers	1 Laughing Cow Light cheese wedge plus 2 FiberRich crackers 1 cup of cut-up red peppers 100-calorie mini bag of light popcorn with Tabasco sauce
Pizza night: 2 slices of thin-crust cheese pizza (2 Angel Carbs) Small mixed green salad with light oil and vinegar dressing 1 light beer 1 cup berries	*Out for sushi dinner:* Small green salad with 2 T dressing Miso soup Oshitashi 5 pieces sashimi 1 yellowtail scallion roll (or other nonfried, nonspicy sushi roll) 2 light beers	*Cooking at home:* 8 oz homemade chicken parm lite (see recipe page 275) with 1½ cups steamed or lightly sautéed spinach plus 1 package of shirataki 1 glass of wine 1 cup of berries

Male Three-Week Sample Menus

	Monday: VOLUME-CONTROLLED RECOVERY DAY	Tuesday	Wednesday	Thursday
Breakfast	0% or 2% Greek yogurt with ½ cup Kashi Go Lean and 1 sliced banana	*Breakfast on-the-go:* Gnu bar Apple Grande skim latte	*Homemade smoothie:* 6 oz plain or 0% Greek yogurt, ice, 1 T ground flaxseed, 1 cup frozen berries, 1 t natural peanut butter plus 1 serving of protein powder	*Dunkin' Donuts:* Eggwhite veggie flatbread Coffee with skim milk
Lunch	*From deli:* Turkey sandwich on 2 slices whole-wheat bread with raw veggies (lettuce/ tomato/ cucumbers/ sprouts) and mustard, and 1 slice of cheese or avocado	*Order into office:* Grilled chicken kabob with grilled peppers, onions, tomatoes, 2 T Tzatziki sauce	*Lunch meeting:* Turkey sandwich (3 oz grilled chicken with lettuce, tomato and mustard on whole wheat bread plus 3 more oz chicken out of 2nd sandwich (no bread) with a side mixed green salad (no croutons and 1 T salad dressing)	*Out for lunch:* 2 appetizers: Caprese salad (1 thick slice or 2 thin slices mozzarella plus tomato) Steamed mussels in white wine or garlic broth
Snack	Kind bar	2 FiberRich crackers and 1 Laughing Cow light cheese and 1 peach	NuGo bar	1 fruit
Dinner	*Frozen dinner:* Trader Joe's chicken tikka masala 2 cups of steamed vegetables Fruit	*Mexican dinner out:* 2 T guacamole with sliced jicama (no chips) Grilled chicken or shrimp fajita, no tortilla, no rice, all of the sautéed onions and peppers and ½ cup black beans 2 vodka sodas with lime	*Pick up from market:* 6 oz turkey meatloaf Side of brussels sprouts (1 cup) Small side of edamame succo-tash (3 oz)	*Frozen dinner:* Amy's single serve margherita pizza (400 calories) Plus mixed green salad with 1 T oil and vinegar 1 orange

Friday	Saturday	Sunday
Thomas Light whole-grain English muffin with 180-calorie packet of Justin's nut butter and ½ sliced banana	2 frozen Van's organic or Kashi Go Lean waffles with ½ cup 1% whipped cottage cheese plus ½ cup blueberries (1 t light syrup optional)	*Making eggs at home for brunch:* Homemade egg sandwich: Morning Star sausage patty on light whole-grain English muffin with 2 scrambled eggs and 1 slice of low-fat cheese
Chopped green salad with lean protein: mixed greens and 3 nonstarchy raw veggies, double protein (grilled chicken, turkey, egg whites, tofu, salmon, shrimp, dry tuna) with balsamic vinegar and 1 T olive oil 2 FiberRich crackers	*Subway lunch:* Subway 6-inch wheat roll with double sliced turkey or chicken, lettuce, tomato, mustard and one slice cheese 1 light yogurt 1 pack of apple slices	
2 FiberRich crackers and 1 Babybel light cheese wheel	Kopali Organics Superfoods mix Later snack: 1 fruit	100-calorie container of hummus with 2 FiberRich crackers and cut-up raw veggies Later snack: 1 fruit Later snack: 2–3 slices of turkey or 1 piece of ostrich jerky
Steakhouse dinner: 2 glasses of wine Tomato and red onion salad (with 2 T vinaigrette or balsamic vinegar) 10 oz filet mignon A few spoonfuls of shared vegetable sides: sautéed mushrooms and steamed broccoli Shared fruit plate	*Ordering in Thai:* 1 cup tom yum soup 2 pieces of chicken satay Small green papaya salad (no meat) 6 oz chicken or shrimp with vegetables in chili basil sauce (no rice)	*Cooking at home:* Angel Chicken Paillard (see recipe page 274): 8 oz chicken plus add sautéed mushrooms and 1 fist of brown rice or sweet potato 1 light beer 17 frozen grapes

Create Your Shopping List

Now that you've seen the Blueprint and you're familiar with the sample menus, it will be helpful to jot down some of the meals that appeal to you for your week ahead. Then you can create a shopping list that will guide you as you stock up on some essentials. It makes such a difference to be prepared; you don't want to find yourself standing in front of the fridge at 8:00 P.M. one night with nothing planned for dinner! And be sure to check out my complete shopping list on page 278. I've tried all the foods I'm recommending, and they include many terrific suggestions from my clients. (If you find a great food choice that you love, tweet it to me at @heatherbauer_rd.)

Here's a sample shopping list. It will supply you with a few breakfasts, some brown-bag lunches and some frozen dinners. Obviously, yours will reflect your tastes and lifestyle.

➤ 0% fat free 6 oz Fage Greek yogurt

➤ 2% Breakstone's 4 oz pack cottage cheese

➤ Eggs

➤ 4 ¼-lb bags of fresh turkey

➤ Fiber-rich crackers

➤ Gnu bars

➤ Kashi Go Lean cereal

➤ Amy's Light & Lean frozen meals

➤ Columbia River Organics frozen broccoli and string beans

➤ Organic chicken breasts

➤ Arnold 100-calorie sandwich thins

➤ Dr. Praeger's California Veggie Burgers

➤ Organic Valley reduced-fat shredded cheese

➤ Cucina Antica marinara sauce

➤ Tofu shirataki noodles

➤ Earthbound Farms boxed arugula

➤ Tomatoes

➤ Berries

➤ Pink Lady apples

Tweaking the Blueprint

Everyone has different weight loss goals and different Diet Devils. We all need some personal attention when it comes to making a diet the perfect plan. I wish I could sit down with you for an hour and comb through your issues and make adjustments to this diet so it will suit you to a T. Since I can't do that let's look at a few adjustments that you might want to consider in the basic Blueprint to make it fit you like a glove.

KNOW YOUR DEVILS   This is one of the main points of this book and one of the main lessons I've learned in years of weight loss counseling: Know yourself. Take my quiz, identify your Devils and learn from the advice I give on how to conquer each one later in the book.

MEN VERSUS WOMEN   The first big difference in dieters, as in life, is men versus women. Pay attention to these differences when you're tweaking the Blueprint to fit you. Learn the differences if you're dieting with your spouse. As far as losing weight is concerned, my female clients tend to do better focusing on calories. It's generally harder for women to lose weight and they need to pay more attention to fine-tuning their diet. Small changes seem to be more important for women, and careful attention to their food journal will pay dividends in weight loss success.

Men, on the other hand, tend to lose weight more easily. Their big issue is typically volume. Calories matter of course for men, but fat doesn't seem to be as much of a negative in their diets. Men can get away with more calories, more fat, and relatively more volume. When women have a frozen dinner, it's usually enough for them; men will often need additional veggie sides to help fill them up.

How Much Weight Do You Have to Lose?

If You Have Twenty Pounds or More to Lose

Your primary focus is cutting out Devil Carbs and sticking with the right amount of healthy carbs. Everything else will fall into place after that. Don't worry too much about the fat, protein volume and so on. You need to go to the higher range of volume when you follow the Blueprint. Cut out the Devil Carbs *entirely* but go for greater volume on your salads, veggies and protein. That will help you feel full and satisfied right from the very beginning. If you start too small with your food choices, you'll be hungry. So, for example, you'd have two carbs a day rather than one and a higher number of fruits. You'd need more protein and more veggies at each meal to stay satisfied. With a frozen dinner, you're going to want a side of veggies and you can have a higher calorie range at dinner. I also suggest that if you're not exercising already, wait to begin. Lose your first ten or fifteen pounds before you consider beginning to exercise. Focus on your food. It's too much to try to tackle both at once. Once you lose those first important pounds and you're comfortable with the Blueprint, it will be much easier to begin an exercise routine. You'll be much more likely to stick with it because you'll have your healthy momentum working for you and you'll feel more in control. Be sure to check out the Hungry Order suggestions I've included in "Dine Out Devils Survival Guide" (page 228).

If You Have Five to Ten Pounds to Lose

Many clients come to me as educated diet veterans. They're eating fewer carbs and they've cut out most of their Devil Carbs. But they still can't lose weight. Their problem is most often volume. They need to reduce the amount of food they eat. Of course it's not always so simple because often they have Diet Devils that are prompting them to consume more than they even know. But, in general, if you have fewer pounds to lose you're going to downsize your volume. Go from a sub to a sandwich. Go from a Chinese carryout meal (even a healthy one of steamed veggies and protein) to a frozen dinner. Go from a bag of baby carrots to a 130-calorie Gnu bar. Up your good carbs and downsize volume. Be scrupulous with your food journal and review it carefully to find the Devils that may be haunting you. Pay closer attention to fat intake; cut it down to boost weight loss. Be sure to check out the Lean Order recommendations I've included in "Dine Out Devils Survival Guide" (page 228).

What's Worked for You in the Past?

If you're a veteran dieter and have been on a number of diets you know that some worked better for you than others, even if none of them were totally effective. Which worked best? A low-carb diet? Weight Watchers? Nutrisystem? Look at the features of that diet that were especially helpful to you and tweak BID in that direction. For example, if a low-carb diet worked better for you in the past, you may want to think about skipping an Angel Carb every other day. You don't need to have carbs every day: You can skip some days if you want. If you're on track with your crackers, cereal or oatmeal plus your fruit, you're getting enough fiber and carbs. Some clients tell me Weight Watchers was relatively good for them. They like to have a pizza now and again, a sandwich at lunch and brown rice at dinner. Weight Watchers includes many more carbs than a low-carb plan, so if this diet was helpful, carbs are probably not a big issue for you. You can allow a bit more variety and flexibility. Of course you still have to watch volume and you still have to beat your Devils. For some people weight loss plans like Jenny Craig, Nutrisystem or Zone, which include a packaged delivery of food, have worked best for them in the past. Clients will tell me that they lost weight on one of these systems, but afterward, when they started eating in the real world, the weight came back. This is the main problem with these plans. For people who've been successful on the packaged-food plans, volume control is a big issue. They have to be meticulous about portion sizes. Frozen dinners two or three times a week for dinner and once or twice for lunch are very helpful.

Your Little Black Food Book

I know you're eager to begin to actually diet, but there's just one more thing I want to share with you. Here's a key question I ask clients when I meet with them for the first time: *Are you willing to write down what you eat?* As someone who's worked with hundreds of people who are trying to lose weight, I know that if you are not willing to keep a basic food journal, your chances of success are reduced. It's not just my experience that tells me a food journal works: Quite a number of studies have *proven* that people who keep notes on what they eat are far more successful at achieving permanent weight loss.

Now, by "food journal" I don't mean a complicated, detailed, obsessive volume. Your food journal should be anything that works for you. *Simple* and *organized* is crucial. My clients have had success with anything from a little drugstore assignment pad to a BlackBerry. Some of my clients love to record what they've eaten in apps like the one available at loseit.com. Others have told me that the apps are too complicated and frustrating to use. If you're in the latter camp, don't stress yourself: You don't need the ounces and the recipes for what you're eating; keep it simple.

When you first begin keeping a food journal, it's important to write down as many details as you can. As time goes by, you can streamline your journal to be short and sweet, but it's important to first see what you are eating and when. Besides writing down all that you eat, you might want to note in your journal how hungry you were when you ate—especially if it was a snack. This helps you pay attention to your personal appetite fluctuations and how they affect your eating. Your journal will also be the best tool for identifying and tracking your Devils. For instance, if you ate a sleeve of crackers after an upsetting phone call you might want to make note of that. You want all significant information about your eating habits in black and white at first—it will help you figure out which Devils you need to concentrate on.

On pages 68 and 69 are sample blank food journal pages that you can copy or use as a template for your own journal. I usually suggest that you fill out your journal in the evening, before bed. That seems to work best for most people. Some people make notes in the course of the day and that works too. But keep up with your notes on a daily basis: If you skip a day

Food Journal

	Monday	Tuesday	Wednesday
Breakfast *			
Lunch			
Snack			
Dinner			
Water			
Exercise			
Triumphs			
Dirty Deeds			

*For those who need a mid-morning snack, insert here:

Thursday	Friday	Saturday	Sunday

Goals:

1. _____

2. _____

3. _____

or two you may find that you have no idea what you ate forty-eight hours ago!

How detailed do you need to be about the food itself? Not terribly. It's sufficient to say, for example, "yogurt and banana" for breakfast, "chicken Caesar salad" for lunch and "chicken breast, broccoli, baked potato, 1 glass of wine" for dinner. Some of my veteran dieter clients have kept a food diary in the past and they sometimes are inclined to be more detailed. This makes sense if you're a veteran or if you are having trouble losing weight even after you've followed my program for two weeks. If that's the case, it could well be that portion control is an issue for you and that you need to spend more time on the details of your diary. If you only have a few pounds to lose—say five to ten—then it's good to be more detailed in your notes, about both portions and ingredients (for example, what type of dressing you had on your salad, how many ounces of protein were in your meal, how many calories were in your frozen dinner). For more guidance on this, see "Plateaus and Tune-Up Techniques" (page 249).

You'll notice that I have an entry in the journal for your Triumphs. Your Triumphs are your successes. Perhaps you reached your water goal. Perhaps you passed up the breadbasket at dinner. Perhaps you got in a good hour of exercise. Log all this in your Triumphs.

You'll see another entry for what I call Dirty Deeds. Years ago when I first asked my clients to create food journals and bring them to our meetings, I was surprised to see that so few of them were guilty of the little picks and tastes that most people indulge in. But when I began to dig a little deeper I learned that yes, many of them were filching fries from their kids' plates and grabbing candies from their accountants' desks. But they were not recording it because they knew they shouldn't do it and they didn't know exactly *how* to record it. So I created Dirty Deeds. Dirty Deeds is a category in your journal that allows you to record any missteps. A planned treat, like a bite of your child's birthday cake, is not a Dirty Deed. An unplanned treat, like licking the frosting off the rest of the cake, is a Dirty Deed.

Keep track of your water intake. This is important. It's going to make a big difference in your success. Also include any alcohol here.

And if you're getting exercise, log that too. Some people like to put down lots of detail on their exercise (distance covered, time); others simply note, say, "45-minute walk." Either is fine.

How long do you need to keep a food journal? I recommend one full month. Research says it takes about three weeks to change a habit (which is why I'm giving you a twenty-one-day Blueprint) so this gives you a nice margin of error to create a new habit. Most of my clients continue to keep a journal sporadically. It's a very helpful reminder. Many people have told me that they use their food journals until they reach their weight loss goal. Then, if they feel a pound or two creeping up, they go right back to making their evening notes. You'll see: Keeping track of what you eat is going to help you stick to your healthy eating plan.

One more word to newbie food journalists: Be honest! No one is peeking at this journal but you, and it's not going to be graded. It all counts. Even if the calories in what you ate are negligible, just making a note of the food in your journal will help you find important patterns. Remember, it's not just about calories. It's also about the types of food you eat, when you eat them and, for many people, how you feel when you eat.

After a week, set aside some time to study your journal. It's going to be a super effective tool for helping you to examine your actual diet and figuring out your Diet Devils. So, scan your days: Where are your trouble spots? Most people will see trends. Do you do a lot of eating at night, after dinner? You may be bedeviled by the Late-Night Shuffle. Do you eat out a lot? Could be you've got to focus on your Dine-Out Devil. Are you eating a healthy breakfast and lunch but just picking off your kids' plates for dinner? Do you skip breakfast but overeat at lunch? Are there any emotional patterns to your eating? Do you tend to snack when you're bored?

Sample Food Journal

Rita, one of my clients, recently quit her job and, with her second child off to college, is struggling with an empty nest and a lack of schedule. This is one of her first entries:

Breakfast: coffee w/milk, yogurt, banana

Snack: ½ English muffin w/butter (leftover from husband's breakfast; mindless snacking!)

Lunch: tuna sandwich, apple (not really that hungry; could have skipped the apple)

Afternoon snack: bowl of popcorn—not the healthy kind— but I was hungry. Got a call at 7:00 P.M.: hubby's going to be late. I'm starving: five Ritz crackers, three with cheddar

Dinner: at home with husband—starving! Homemade pasta Bolognese, small salad, 1 pc bread; 2 glasses red wine; another pc bread while cleaning up

TV snack: more popcorn watching TV; another glass red wine (hubby was having more and I wanted to be social)

Dirty Deed: 2 small chocolate samples & one small paper cup of granola while food shopping

Exercise: Ugh. Never got to that.

And her food journal in her second week of the Blueprint:

> *Breakfast:* coffee w/milk, Greek yogurt, berries
>
> *Snack:* tea (surprisingly, it filled me up!)
>
> *Lunch:* (with friends) chicken Caesar salad, light balsamic dressing (no bread!); decaf skim cappuccino
>
> *Afternoon snack:* 2 FiberRich crackers with Babybel cheese (definitely helps keep me full till dinner)
>
> *Dinner:* Amy's frozen veggie lasagna, 2 stalks of leftover broccoli, 1 glass red wine (husband on business trip; now I'm always trying to "go frozen" when he's gone!)
>
> *Water:* 7 cups—almost to my goal
>
> *Exercise:* Coaxed a friend into a 45-minute exercise walk this morning

Comparing the two different entries, you can see that Rita made a few simple changes to get things under control. Her original journal showed that her eating wasn't terrible, but it was definitely not going to promote weight loss. Writing it all down helped her really focus on her food and on changing behaviors.

Recovery Strategies That Will Save Your Diet

Among the most important and effective tools for permanent weight loss, in addition to your food journal, are my recovery strategies. Most of us tend toward the ambitious when it comes to weight loss plans. (Who can resist the diet that promises

Jean's Journal

I was totally dismayed when Heather told me that it was important to keep a food journal. I don't even like to keep a shopping
list! But she said it was a deal breaker so I forced myself into it.
I got a small red notebook and kept it in my pocket. Once
I started, I realized keeping the journal made me pay much
more attention to what I was eating. Sometimes the mere idea
that I would have to later record my indulgence would be
enough to stop me from going overboard. I also noticed that I
was most likely to have a little mindless binge in the late afternoon. So Heather suggested that I simply plan a snack for 4:00
P.M. What a difference that made! I kept my journal the whole
time until I got to my goal, which took about ten months. Now I
pull it out if I feel like I'm backsliding.

you'll lose ten pounds in a week?) But most of those plans involve deprivation and restriction so it's almost impossible to
stick to them. That's where my recovery strategies come in.
Everyone who struggles to lose weight needs to discover how
to climb back up from a fall. You know what I'm talking about.
Almost everyone who has tried to lose weight has failed, at
least once. You start a new diet with boundless enthusiasm.
You lose a few pounds in the first week and, whoo hoo! Life is
good. But then, ka boom! Something makes you lose control
and overeat. I was once left alone in the back of a cab with a
box of a half dozen fantastic cupcakes. (Only my food journal
knows the ending to that story but I promise you, it wasn't
pretty.) Almost every single client I've ever had has been able
to tell me about his or her diet failures and how they came
about. And for almost all of these people, these failures became a brick wall at the end of their diet road. Demoralized
and totally discouraged, they gave up and typically regained
the weight they'd lost plus a few pounds.

Here's how to put a stop to the food hangovers that mess up your head and your resolve. Recognize that if you change your mind you will change your weight. The most important step you can take toward weight loss success is simply to make a resolution that, despite any lapses, you are going to stick with the diet. Close your eyes and repeat three times: "Nothing is a diet breaker!" Rather than thinking in terms of a temporary goal—fitting into a dress or a bathing suit—it's much more effective to develop a long-term goal: *think in terms of becoming a healthy eater.* That's a lifetime goal. When you set your sights on the long term, you can recover more quickly from any missteps. Think like this and you will no longer be the victim of any of the diet mistakes that used to send you into a tailspin. Because nothing is a diet breaker!

So how do you achieve this nirvana? You learn my recovery strategies. These strategies work because they are not weird, extreme measures. Many of my clients have told me how they have tried fasts, juice cleanses and skipping meals after a binge. These efforts tend to set you up for failure while my recovery strategies keep you on the track of clean, healthy, three-meal-a-day living. They're simple; they're structured; they work. Here are the three most effective techniques my clients have used to bounce back from a diet fail:

➤ A Protein Day

➤ A Volume-Controlled Day

➤ A Veggie Night

A PROTEIN DAY A Protein Day is the major reset tool used by my clients. It's great for the day after a major calorie overload or any serious Plunge. It's also terrific for the day after you've returned from a trip. It's a simple tool that gets you back into the action without delay. A Protein Day is just what it sounds like: a day in which your diet is primarily protein. It's a clean, simple meal plan that helps reset your body.

Here are the meal options for a Protein Day:

➤ Breakfast: 4–6 egg white vegetable omelet or 2 hard-boiled eggs. (for those who don't eat eggs: 3 oz poached chicken or 3 oz tofu)

➤ Lunch: 3–6 oz of grilled chicken over mixed greens with balsamic vinegar, 1 t olive oil and lemon for flavor; raw cucumbers and mushrooms can be added

➤ Optional snack: 1 orange, 2 clementines or ½ banana (males can add ¼ pound turkey if hungry)

➤ Dinner: 3–6 oz of grilled chicken, fish or lean sirloin, mixed green salad with balsamic vinegar, 1 t oil and 1 cup steamed veggies (men can have unlimited veggies and upper limit of protein)

➤ No snack; no dairy; no alcohol

A VOLUME-CONTROLLED DAY Want to recover from an unfortunate evening—perhaps a party or a pizza binge—and give your diet brain a rest at the same time? A Volume-Controlled Day is for you. I came up with it as an alternative to the Protein Day. Some clients know that they just won't be able to get through a Protein Day. If this describes you, then go for the Volume-Controlled Day. The "control" refers to portion control. So a Volume-Controlled Day is simply one in which all your meals are portion controlled. It helps you get your volume back on track, recenters you and gets you back to three healthy meals a day. What could be easier? No thinking; no overeating!

Here's an example of a Volume-Controlled Day menu:

➤ Breakfast: 0%–2% Greek yogurt (8 oz container), ¼ cup Kashi Go Lean, 1 apple

➤ Lunch: 2 slices light wheat bread, 4 slices turkey, lettuce, tomato, mustard (men can have additional 2 oz protein and 1 slice of avocado)

➤ Optional snack: 1 apple or 1 orange or 1 small banana

➤ Dinner: any frozen dinner on my shopping list (page 62), under 400 calories for men and under 300 calories for women (men can add steamed green veggies); if you're eating out, have a baked potato with salsa and mustard and two sides of steamed green veggies

➤ No dairy; no alcohol; 8–10 cups water

Clients will sometimes tell me that they can't do a Protein Day or a Volume-Controlled Day because they're not eating at home. This is not a valid excuse! You can actually eat every meal out and have a successful recovery day. Breakfast can be anywhere (diner, deli, restaurant) that you can find a granola bar for under 180 calories and a hand fruit or an egg white omelet. Your lunch might be a chicken Caesar salad with no croutons and parmesan and with balsamic vinegar dressing or an under-400-calorie sandwich from Subway or Starbucks. And almost any restaurant can serve you a mixed green salad, any grilled protein and a steamed or sautéed veggie for dinner. Simple, no?

A VEGGIE NIGHT A Veggie Night is another excellent recovery technique. In my experience, a Veggie Night will appeal particularly to women as a recovery technique, although some male clients can also find it effective if they make sure that the volume of the meal is satisfying. A Veggie Night can be especially useful on a weekend or Monday night when you want to get a head start on your diet week. Some clients build in a Veggie Night to their weekly menus just as a matter of routine. Veggie Nights are also for those times when you get home very late and you just want something simple and fast to satisfy you before bed.

A Veggie Night is just what you'd guess: a night when your dinner is simply vegetables. The Veggie Night dinner is a baked white or sweet potato and 2 measured cups of steamed vegetables. The vegetables can be any vegetable of your choice from the Blueprint. Since you can microwave both the potato and the vegetables, your dinner can be ready in less than ten minutes. There are now several brands of plain vegetables on the market that you can steam in just a few minutes in the bag they come in. Check my shopping list for a good selection of brand-name, quick-prep veggies.

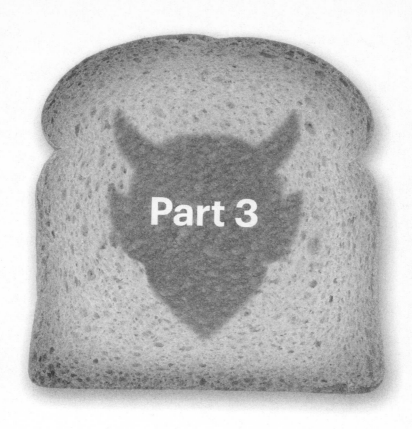

Part 3

Taming Your Diet Devils

As I discussed in the introduction, most of us dieters have Diet Devils—moments, situations, or emotions—that make shedding those pounds even harder. Now that you have the basic diet to follow, it's time to learn the techniques you'll need to finally and permanently tame those Devils and get you on the road to successful weight loss. You've also already identified your personal Devils: Some of you have only a couple of Devils; others may have all ten. Whatever your situation, read through your Devils and start to adopt the techniques. These strategies, coupled with the Blueprint, will help you tailor the most effective diet program you've ever tried.

Note: Most people will need to read about the FreeStyle Devil since that one plagues just about every dieter who's ever tried and failed to reach a weight loss goal. So read FreeStyle first and then move on to the Devils that emerged when you took the quiz at the beginning of the book.

Diet Devil #1
Free-Style Dieting

Most of my clients are what I call veteran dieters. They've been on diets numerous times. They're sophisticated about food and weight loss, and they know about portion control, carbs, cleanses, glycemic index, the whole shebang. They're vegans, pescetarians, lacto-ovo vegetarians, and pesco-lacto-ovo vegetarians. In fact, one of my clients recently told me she's a "dietarian." It's all "been there, done that" as far as they're concerned. So when they find themselves dipping into the "fat" section of their closets they decide they're going to get a grip on things. Maybe they'll cut out desserts or bread or pasta. They'll skip the bedtime pint of Häagen-Dazs, actually walk the dog instead of letting him run out and use the backyard, and maybe they'll try to cut down on their drinking. They decide to "really watch what they eat." I call this the Free-Style Devil. No specific plan, just a renewed effort to get control and shed some weight.

Sounds good, right? You may have tried this yourself more than once. If so, I bet you've discovered that this approach rarely succeeds. Usually by the end of the first week of the Free-Style Devil you're right back where you started because "something came up"—a party, a dinner out, a trip, a bowl of M&M's on someone's desk. Or you watch what you eat but you don't realize that you're eating portions big enough for two or three. Or maybe you have some outdated diet rules in your head like "eliminate all fat," or enjoy "healthy snacks" like a handful of nuts twice a day. Often you simply get tired of paying attention. We all crave adventure: cutting back on alcohol and fat is no adventure. In short, the usual pattern for the Free-Style Devil is that your old habits—your personal Diet Devils—suck you back into the world of pudge.

Free-Style is a subtle Devil: It seems like a really good idea but it seduces you into wasting time with vague resolutions that will never get you to your goal.

The simple fact is, *without a plan and a real commitment to lose, it's very difficult to be successful at long-term weight loss.*

Effective weight loss is all about structure. Not "you must eat this; you must not eat that" structure, but rather simple rules about eating that give you a clear picture every day of what you're going to eat. Too much decision making, too much uncertainty, too much wondering how to handle tough eating challenges all lead you astray. One of my clients once said to me, "I really want to lose weight and I think I know what I should eat, but I just can't do it." That's because this client had so many vague ideas in her head about weight loss that she couldn't settle down and put her desire into action. If you are serious about losing weight you have to have a plan, Stan. And you have to commit to it. So let's banish the Free-Style Devil once and for all. There are three important strategies that help create a structure for your diet and free you from the Free-Style Dieting Devil.

1. Use Your Food Journal

I've discussed your food journal on page 68. It's a simple concept but so powerful: Writing down what you eat helps you keep track of what you're actually putting in your mouth. It's a window into your own eating habits and routines and, if you record faithfully, it will help you see patterns in your eating and—by helping to identify your Devils—find solutions to the eating patterns that have led you astray in the past.

2. Embrace Phase Eating

Phase Eating is a very powerful weight loss strategy—simply eat the same healthy breakfast, lunch, or dinner day after day for a stretch of time. Many people—including many of my clients—find that choosing one or two favorite breakfasts and lunches gets them easily through their diet week. In fact, quite a number of clients have told me that they've been discouraged in the past by diets with too many food selections. However, I wouldn't recommend repeating the same dinner too frequently, with the possible exception of occasionally repeating your favorite frozen dinners. Dinner should be a pleasurable part of your day and something to look forward to, so I recommend that you use Phase Eating primarily for breakfast and lunch. You'll notice that my Blueprint relies on Phase Eating. Clients have told me that Phase Eating has "given them permission" to take a lot of the obsession with food out of their daily lives. Don't you agree that the less you think about food, the easier it is to eat better and eat less?

3. Rely on Recovery Strategies

You'll find a complete description of my recovery strategies in the previous chapter on page 73. I mention them again here because they're critical to your diet success. To refresh your memory, here are the strategies that will banish your mistakes and get you back on track and moving quickly toward your goal weight:

A Protein Day

A Volume-Controlled Day

A Veggie Night

Rachael's Confession

I used to be totally obsessed with what I ate. When my weight was up, I felt guilty and was always thinking about what I should eat next and worrying about whether I'd make a good choice. And whether I'd feel guilty after I ate. It was insane. When Heather told me to "Phase Eat" it was almost like a weight was lifted off my shoulders (as well as my hips)! I picked a healthy breakfast that I knew I could happily eat every morning, a lunch that I could put on mental speed dial, and then a few frozen dinners that I could stock up on. Done. It's heaven. Now that 90% of my brain is not filled with agonizing about meals I'm free to live my life. Of course I switch things up now and again but the heavy lifting is done.

Diet Devil #2
The Plunge

"One Bite Is Too Many; a Thousand Is Not Enough"

f there were one Diet Devil that seems to plague almost all of my clients, it's the Plunge. The Plunge is your biggest weight loss enemy and my guess is that if you're reading this book, you've experienced it. Call it what you will, a diet collapse, a binge, a lost day. . . . My clients may have different names for it, but they all recognize it as a very, very bad thing.

A Plunge is not about having a little piece of chocolate at a party. It's not about sneaking your hand into your friend's popcorn box at the movies. It's an all-out freaking total descent into the food abyss. It's an empty bag of honey wheat pretzels, the frosting scraped off the top of the cake, four bowls of Frosted Flakes with skim milk. One recent study found that participants who succumbed to a chocolate truffle and ate it were more eager to continue on with ice cream, pizza and potato chips. Folks who resisted the truffle were better able to resist other subsequent treats. Well, duh. Most of us know from experience that one truffle almost always leads to another. In fact, my clients describe their experience with the Plunge as a sort of out-of-body experience. "I hardly remember ripping open the bag of chips and before I knew it they were all gone," or "I was just going to have a bite of the cupcake and suddenly I'd eaten all four of them." What's worse is that the Plunge can often team up with many of the other Devils like Celebrations, Dine-Out, and Emotional Eating, doubling its danger.

So put down that Butterfinger and take a closer look at what's really happening here. Say you had a total Plunge at Whole Foods. You were buying some healthy salad greens and vegetables for yourself and then picking up a few things for the kids and the bag of kettle corn landed in your basket and on the way home you ripped it open and ate it and when you went into the house to get a wipe for the now-sticky steering wheel you figured, what the heck, and you reached into the fridge and polished off that last slice of cake. And now you're eyeing the crusts the kids left in the pizza box on the counter. Well, go ahead and finish those crusts. And here's about how many calories you will have consumed by the time you regain your senses: anywhere from 500 to 800 calories, so let's call it even at 650 calories. Yes, you made a mistake. Yes, you're feeling disgusted with yourself and, come to think about it, a little sick. But, when all is said and done, you've made a 650-calorie mistake. Is it worth throwing away a week or a month of effort for 650 calories? Of course not!

Here's the single most important thing to know about the Plunge: *The worst part is not the calories—it's the way the Plunge messes with your head.* Because you were doing well. You'd built up some diet cred. This time was going to be different. And now you'd gone and blown it. Or so the voice in your head tells you. You're hopeless, the devilish voice whispers, you'll never lose any weight. So you believe that voice and give up, maybe for the second or third or fourth time. Or maybe you just keep saying to yourself, "I'll start tomorrow." But the backlog of bad feelings robs you of any real incentive to take your resolutions seriously.

So . . . I won't tell you not to have a Plunge. You're never going to *plan* to have one. But I will share some effective strategies you can use to cope with the devastating aftereffects of a Plunge and also some strategies that could help you dodge one next time around.

Before we even explore the depths of the dreaded Plunge and how one finds oneself at the bottom of that abyss, I want to throw some cold water on you and share two significant tips that might just change your eating future.

Post-Plunge Recovery

The most important strategy following a Plunge is to simply get back up on the healthy horse. But before I give you my strategies for how to avoid almost all Plunges, I'm going to tell you how to recover from a Plunge. You probably have already read about my recovery strategies (page 73), but sometimes with a Plunge you need something more *immediate* to reset your clock and get your head back in the right place. Even as you are wiping the crumbs from your lap and wondering what hit you, it's time to begin your post-Plunge recovery. First, and most important, don't dwell on your lapse. Don't tell yourself what a failure you are and don't beat yourself with all that blah, blah, blah about how you can't ever lose weight, etc., etc. Rather, do something *active* to wash the Plunge away and get your mind back in the healthy groove. Pick your strategy:

➤ A clean meal
➤ A water flush

A clean meal is just what it sounds like. If you had a Plunge in the morning or afternoon, your next meal should be clean— that is, made up of a protein and a vegetable. That's it. No carb.

No alcohol. No questions. Your initial thought after a Plunge may be to just skip your next meal entirely, but this is a mistake. Eat a meal, but make it clean. If you had a nighttime Plunge, follow it up the next morning with a clean breakfast, which is two hard-boiled eggs or an egg white omelet or 3 ounces of turkey or tofu. You're not going to mind it because you're probably full from your Plunge and you're ready to make amends.

A *water flush* is a quick and effective Plunge penance. This is just what you think it is. As soon as you realize that you've just Plunged, drink a liter—4 cups, or 32 ounces—of water. Yes, you're already full but this will help your body process all the salt or sugar you just consumed and while it feels uncomfortable initially, you will see that it's a great strategy for getting back on track. It also almost guarantees that you will not go back to the kitchen for more food, because you won't be able to fit one more bite in your tummy. A bedtime Plunge? Do the water flush anyhow: You may have to get up a few times during the night but you'll feel much better than you otherwise would have in the morning. And you'll start the new day with your Plunge far behind you.

What Plungers Need to Know

Here are the strategies that will help you avoid future Plunges.

Break the plunge cycle by allowing yourself 1–2 angel carbs a day

Diets that eliminate whole food groups or are extreme in any way are the worst for Plungers because the inevitable failures they cause can trigger plunges. Many Plungers live in a black-and-white world of either gluttony or starvation. Perhaps you've said this to yourself in the past: "I'm never going to eat another bagel," but once you do eat another bagel you fall into a hopeless plunge. Successful dieters need to learn to live in a nuanced world. On my Blueprint you're allowed 1–2 Angel carbs every day. You can even enjoy a sandwich if you like as one of those Angel carbs. Seeing that you can lose weight while allowing yourself carb choices can be incredibly freeing for a plunger. Remember too that there's no "perfect" on this plan: if you eat something you hadn't planned on, like a Devil Carb, just call it a carb and move on.

EMBRACE FINITE FOOD If you're vulnerable to the Plunge, you will find that Finite Food is your friend. What is it? It's food with an ending. It's fruit that fits in your hand like an apple or an orange, not fruit you have to count out like grapes or cherries. It's single-portion frozen dinners, not a whole rotisserie chicken and a huge salad. It's a ½-cup container of cottage cheese, versus a four-serving container. It's portion-controlled snacks and any healthy, prepackaged, single-serve food: one with a healthy, diet-friendly limit built in. These Finite Foods help you keep portions in control and help protect you from a Plunge. Finite Food is the opposite of poppable, pickable, unstoppable foods—like pretzels, chips, popcorn, grapes, even cherry tomatoes—that you can read about in "Boredom Bingeing." Those kinds of foods are the enemy for Plungers. But Finite Food brings you back to the land of happy, healthy eating.

KNOW YOUR TRIGGER FOODS I have never yet had a client who binges on turkey, fish, vegetables or fruit. No one has ever sat in my office and with downcast eyes admitted, "Yes, I ate the whole bowl of brussels sprouts." When you are lured into the Plunge it's always because of one of your trigger foods:

something salty or something sweet. Usually it's a big fat carb. You already know your trigger foods. The particular problem with indulging in your trigger food is that it never stops there. You never have one Hershey's Kiss. You have fifteen or twenty. And then move on to whatever else is lying around and then skip dinner. . . . So think about your trigger foods and take a minute to imagine them with big fat dangerous devil horns on them. Keep clear of them. Empty your kitchen, your desk drawer, and your glove compartment of them.

DON'T SACRIFICE: STRATEGIZE!   Many of my clients start out thinking that it's best to always go for the "light" or "diet" meal. They'll pick a salad with dressing on the side. Or two teeny appetizers for dinner. Or they'll deconstruct the menu, creating a whole new entrée by asking the chef to remove nearly every calorie and every bit of flavor from their meal. These seem like smart choices. And they would be, if you didn't go home afterward so hungry that you have a whole pint of ice cream for dessert. I believe that if there's no real food in your food you're setting yourself up for failure. Know yourself. If you have a small salad at lunch and find yourself crazed with hunger in the late afternoon, it's time to rethink your lunch menu. Same with dinner. If you have something light and at 11:00 P.M. are having a major Plunge, stop sacrificing and start strategizing. Add some healthy calories to your meals. For example, you may be better off having a sandwich instead of a salad at lunch if it's going to satisfy you and help you get through until dinner without a Plunge. And believe it or not, it may be smarter for you anyway: A turkey sandwich is about 300 calories, a Cobb salad clocks in at about 800 calories without the bacon and cheese. Same goes at dinner: Choose something that's satisfying. If you're eating out you might do much better with some grilled fish and two veggies than two little appetizers. It's better to consume an extra couple of hundred calories than a cascading 2,000 calories later!

STOP HOOVERING Are you always the first one finished at any dinner party? Do you eat so fast your knife and fork become a cartoon blur of activity? Do you sometimes eat so fast that you're not even sure what you ate? Do you pick off other people's plates? If so, you are a Hooverer. You vacuum up any food that comes your way. And it's important for you to recognize that it's not always about *what* you eat but also about *how* you eat. For some people, Hoovering is a bad mealtime habit, but for others it can precipitate a Plunge. Hoovering is mindless eating at its worst. For one thing, when you speed eat, you usually consume too much. It takes about twenty minutes for your brain to send the signal that you're full. If you finish your meal in three minutes flat, your brain is getting the "stop" sign waaaay too late and you're probably overeating. Do you often feel absolutely stuffed after a meal? That's a sign that you've been either eating too fast or ignoring your brain's "I'm full" message. *So slow down.* Put your fork down between bites. Have a sip of water. In fact, try to drink three glasses of water in the course of a meal. Chew. The longer you chew your food, the fuller you will feel, the sooner you'll stop eating and the fewer calories you'll take in. Pause for some conversation. Enjoy your food. Slow equals mo, when it comes to weight loss.

NEVER GET HUNGRY It always amazes me how many of my new clients will skip or delay meals. They think that this is a good strategy for taking in fewer calories. But it almost always backfires on them, especially if they're vulnerable to the Plunge. If you are a Plunger, the only time you want to experience real hunger is in the morning, when you wake up. Plungers are almost physically unable to handle temptation when they're hungry. We just go insane. If your tummy is growling and a Milky Way walks by, you can't be responsible for your actions. So always, always, plan your eating day. *Never skip a meal.* Phase Eating (page 85) can make this very easy. Know what you're having for breakfast, lunch and dinner. If you need an afternoon snack, be prepared: pack one.

BEWARE THE WANDER   Some of my clients occasionally indulge in what I call "the Wander." The Wander can begin with a small slice of pizza on the way home, and then maybe a stop at a food store that offers an array of free samples—maybe a cube or three or four or six cubes of cheese and a handful (no one is watching) of honey roasted nuts. And, well, maybe you should skip dinner and just have another couple of those little sausage pizza samples. . . . And by the time you arrive home— your pockets filled with toothpicks, tiny napkins and plastic forks and spoons—it's too late: you've done the Wander. Many clients tell me that they know the best spots in their area to hit on a Wander—the Whole Foods and Costcos and specialty markets that serve the best and most abundant samples. Such wandering can set you back an astonishing number of calories and contribute almost nothing to your sense of satisfaction. The solution to the Wander is simple avoidance. Avoid stores that offer free food samples. Or, if you must shop at one, chew gum or pop a breath mint the minute you enter the shop.

RECOGNIZE A CHANGE IN APPETITE   Many people experience appetite shifts in the course of the year. For some people it's seasonal, for others it's hormonal (like PMS). It could be stress related, weather related, or simply a random change in appetite. If you experience an occasional appetite surge, just go with it to some degree and increase your food intake just a bit. Otherwise, if you stick with your portion-controlled frozen dinner despite an extra hearty appetite you might find yourself in the middle of a Plunge at 10:00 P.M. because you're just not satisfied. So if you're feeling extremely hungry for whatever reason nature has thrown at you, make your meals a little more substantial by adding more steamed veggies or a hand fruit for dessert so that you won't be vulnerable to a Plunge.

Some of my clients experience a surge in appetite as they are losing weight and suddenly experience a day or two when they're *starving*. I don't really have any scientific explanation for this. Perhaps it's because the body is saying, "I want more calories!" The key with this type of hunger is to stay on track. Know that this hunger will only last a day or two. Drink extra water, seltzer or herbal tea. Add in an additional fruit snack and boost your protein by an additional couple of ounces at lunch and dinner. Add extra steamed veggies at lunch and dinner. Take whatever healthy steps you need to avoid a Plunge and stick with your permanent weight loss goals.

BREAK THE SNACK CYCLE!   I know, believe me, I know: you just walked in the door, you're still in your coat and you're standing in front of the open refrigerator door, thinking, hmmmm . . . that last piece of pie? That chunk of baking chocolate at the back of the crisper? That frozen pecan raisin bread that could be defrosted in a flash and slathered, while still warm, with some butter? Take a deep breath, close the fridge. Take off your coat. It only takes fifteen minutes for a craving to pass. Make yourself a cup of tea. Wash your face. Clear some of the clutter from the countertops. There. Feel better? When you're about to slide into a Plunge, you have to divert yourself. It's not a huge big deal; it's just breaking the cycle—delaying the moment when the food reaches your lips—until you no longer feel tempted. It works. Try it.

DON'T BE SCALE OBSESSED   Some of my clients feel inclined to weigh themselves after every glass of water and every trip to the bathroom. This is a mistake, especially for Plungers. Your weight is going to fluctuate constantly and isn't always an accurate reflection of your last meal. Some people retain water after a dinner out; some people are slow to lose weight; some people won't shed an ounce and then suddenly drop five pounds. The problem with checking the scale constantly is that if you don't like the number, it can precipitate a Plunge. It's better to weigh yourself just once a week or so. This should be enough to keep you on track.

ALWAYS BRING YOUR "A" GAME   If anxiety, anger and stress prompt you to eat, you may be an Emotional Eater and particularly vulnerable to The Plunge. Check out my strategies for Emotional Eaters (page 113); It's especially important for these types of eaters to always try to stay positive. Don't ever tell yourself that you blew it. When you have a lapse, just give a big fat "oops" and move on. I've had clients come to me so discouraged by past failures and the echoes of so many Plunges that they didn't really believe they could be successful. Changing the tape in their heads was as important as changing their eating habits. They reached their goals, just as you can.

RECOGNIZE PLUNGEABLE MOMENTS   There are situations where the Plunge can be almost inevitable, like shopping while hungry, kids' birthday parties (It's calorie free if only a three-year-old is watching, right?), Halloween, and Thanksgiving—heck, any holiday for that matter. If you do know that you're going to face a potential Plunge, plan for it. If it's just inevitable that you're going to eat a sampling of your child's Halloween candy, then plan a light lunch and dinner. Don't dip into the plastic pumpkin while starving: Have a snack before you confiscate the loot. Same with difficult social situations. Plan ahead for those eating situations that you know are going to be difficult: Never show up starving, and either allow yourself an indulgence or figure out a way to avoid indulging. But try not to tell yourself that you won't eat anything and then turn around and inhale a Carvel cake.

PSEUDO SHOPPING   You tell yourself it's for your husband. Or your daughter. Or your aunt who might stop by any day now even though you haven't seen her in two years and she lives three states away. I'm talking about the box of cookies or the frozen lemon meringue pie or the bag of peanut M&M's that you just tossed with utter conviction into your shopping cart. You may actually believe, for at least a few seconds, that those goodies are for someone else. But by the time you're watching the cashier stuff them in a bag, you know in your heart that no one but you is going to be chowing down on them. This happens with random goodies and also with pseudo party shopping. You're having another couple over for drinks? Better lay in that wheel of Brie, the two pounds of pistachios, the cheese straws and those lovely chocolate mints in case someone is in the mood for something sweet. And when your guests arrive it suddenly seems a bit crazy to put out enough food to feed the whole security line at JFK, so you scarf down as much as possible in the quiet of your kitchen, and then put out a sensible few nibbles. And eat the rest in the next couple of days. Time to look in the mirror, mirror on the wall and ask yourself, Who's the sneakiest shopper of all? The best way to avoid this certain Plunge is to never, ever, ever shop while hungry. Just don't. And when you do food shop, make a list and stick with it. In fact, if you have a real pseudo shopping issue, consider using one of the many popular delivery services if you have one in your area. That way you can do your shopping from home when you're feeling strong.

PLAN YOUR INDULGENCES   Now, I would be the last person to tell you that you can never enjoy a treat again. But a treat should never turn into a Plunge. How can you manage that? Plan ahead. As a general rule, I also advise clients to try to avoid all indulgences early in the day, when they tend to be strong. Save up and indulge, if you must, in the evening. Indulge with friends; indulge with family; avoid indulging in a work situation. I always think it's best to keep your work life and your private life separate and that holds true for food: There's not as much pleasure in having a dessert at a business lunch as there is in enjoying a dessert with a loved one. Never waste calories; always try to indulge with those you love at a happy, relaxed time in your day. (That means no stuffing candy in your pockets to inhale in the empty elevator.) If you are going to indulge remember to go small and stop. That means, have a little bit of something and then call it quits. Keep those words in your head. And of course, you know yourself: if it's going to be impossible to stop, do everything in your power not to start. For more information on indulgences and how to count them, see the Blueprint, on page 27.

MANAGE FOOD GIFTS Clients have told me that a food gift is their worst nightmare. How do you resist something delicious—say a box of chocolates that sweet Auntie Margie sent you? Wouldn't it be really rude not to eat it? Well, no, dear dieter, it wouldn't. Anyone who gives you a food gift is really sending good thoughts your way. So they want for you what you want: to get slim and healthy. They just don't realize how hard you're working to accomplish that goal. So, if necessary, take a tiny bite of the gift, and then off it goes—to another friend, a coworker, the reception desk, an elderly neighbor, the teacher's lounge . . . wherever you will be safe from it. And guess what? Even if you never tasted a morsel you can still write a thank-you note.

Diet Devil #3
The Late-Night Shuffle

I ask my new clients two questions. The first is, "Do you eat at night?" Some just give me a funny look and say, "You mean dinner?" But many more say "Were you watching me?" And then they launch into full confession mode, telling me all about the amazing amounts of food they can habitually consume between 6:00 P.M. and midnight. And how they just can't stop. The second question is, "Are you hungry in the morning?" Those who are *never* hungry in the morning almost always have a night-eating issue.

Welcome to the world of the Late-Night Shuffle.

Here's the typical scenario: You hold it together all day—through breakfast, lunch and even late afternoon—with healthy meals and maybe one small snack. You feel light and clean. Then your busy day is over and you're back in your nest. All the tensions of the day are evaporating and so is your willpower. So you wander through your kitchen from pantry to fridge eating bits and smidges of this and that. A handful of raisins. A few chunks of cheese. Some leftover lasagna. And then you collapse in front of the TV but something is missing. So you dig out that half a bag of pretzels and, ahhhhh, chewing! Take me home.

The Late-Night Shuffle is the epitome of mindless eating. You barely taste the food. You hardly look at it. It's just bite, chew, bite, chew, bite, chew until bedtime. It's not that you haven't tried to stop. It's not that you don't know you should stop. It's that you just can't.

I'm here to tell you that yes, *you can*! The Late-Night Shuffle is a seductive trap. It's soothing; it's pleasurable; it's become part of your regular routine. But there are strategies that will help you break this bad habit and move quickly to your goal weight.

Most people think the issue with night eating is calories. Of course the calories do count—even in the dark. Many of my night-eating clients consume more calories in the few hours between dinner and bedtime than they do all day long. But the calorie bomb is only part of the problem. *The real challenge of late-night eating is that it's habit forming.* That's right: If you're a late-night eater it's not something you indulge in occasionally. My clients who are late-night eaters tell me that they routinely snack—often in front of the TV—from the time they finish dinner until bedtime. Many of them have stockpiles of these midnight snacking foods—popcorn, cereal, leftover takeout meals—and they tell me about how they become anxious when they know the fridge and pantry are totally bare. How will they get through the evening?

An inevitable issue with the Late-Night Shuffle is that the foods you're drawn to tend to be carbs—Devil Carbs. I have never, in all my years of working with thousands of clients, had someone tell me that they overindulge in broccoli in the evening. Devil Carbs are infinitely more tempting. But of course they tend to be high in fat as well as in salt or sugar. And they tend to be "infinite" foods: Once you start it's almost impossible to stop.

Like so many Diet Devils, night eating is a form of relaxation and stress relief. Most of us have lives that are crazy busy, stressed and overscheduled all day long. We rush from activity to appointment to obligation. Meals are a quick break in our overloaded routines, but often the food—its taste and the pleasure of eating—is beside the point. But when we walk in the door in the evening, well, it's finally time to relax. And unfortunately, for many of us, there's nothing more relaxing than a nice chow down. For many people, the Late-Night Shuffle is the way they soothe and reward themselves at the end of the hectic day.

Fatigue plays a big role in prompting the Late-Night Shuffle. You've been on the fast treadmill all day and now you're exhausted. When you're tired, your resistance is down and it's hard to make good decisions. You know how you can start so strong in the morning and then dissolve into a puddle of pudding at 10:00 P.M.? It's normal and natural. It's just not healthy. And it sends you right back to "go" even if you've eaten well all day long.

Late-night eating can also cause you to sleep poorly since your body is busy digesting all those snacks. As I said above, many of the go-to foods that call your name at 9:00 P.M. are sugary carbs. Sugar is a fast-burning energy source that your body wants to use right up, but you're short-circuiting that option because you're lying on the sofa or in bed. What's a body to do? Get a blood sugar high, followed by a crash. And then that same body with the bouncing metabolism stores those sweet calories as fat! You wake up tired and with a food hangover. One more bit of discouraging news: Many of the treats my clients indulge in just before bed contain chocolate. Whether it's a fudge pop, handfuls of chocolate chips or a few scoops of chocolate ice cream, these foods have a secret payload that's going to torture you into the wee hours: caffeine. Most people never think about the caffeine in chocolate. Admittedly, it's not a large amount of caffeine, but it's definitely enough to disrupt your sleep.

Many of my clients who report a late-night snacking habit have never associated their erratic daytime energy levels with their midnight fridge runs. These are the people who skip breakfast because they're not hungry after snacking so much at bedtime. They tend to then overcompensate by eating too much at lunch or dinner. Meanwhile, their blood sugar is peaking and falling at erratic times during the day, making them tired and cranky. One client told me she spent every afternoon at work just waiting for the coffee wagon to come to her floor because she was so tired by 3:30 that she could hardly function. She was desperate for her afternoon caffeine fix to get her through the rest of her day. She never slept well. But once she shifted the pattern of her eating to regular healthy meals at regular times and also eliminated the Late-Night Shuffle, she had sustained energy throughout her day, thanks to her newly stable blood sugar, and she found that for the first time in a long time she slept really well at night.

Here's something else you're going to struggle with if you're a night eater: discouragement. If you eat well all day and then succumb to night eating, you're going to feel like a failure. That repetitive discouragement of not achieving what you set your mind to can be terribly demoralizing. And night eating, as opposed to some of the other Devils, is something that you must cope with virtually every single day. So let's get a grip on this persistent Devil. Once you understand why you're a mid-night muncher and once you learn how you can substitute good habits for this bad one, you'll be so much more successful in your weight loss efforts.

The key to conquering the Late-Night Shuffle is to put an end once and for all to the habit. I've found over the years that the best way to break a bad habit is to substitute a good habit in its place. So I'm going to give you some alternatives to evening munching that will give you a new lease on life. You might well feel slightly odd the first few nights as you abandon

Are You Never Hungry for Breakfast?

If you often skip breakfast because you're just not hungry, you are probably eating too much at night. The Late-Night Shuffle can throw your appetite out of whack and thus your whole healthy eating day. People who are Late-Night Shufflers should pay special attention to their morning hunger. I'm looking for what I call a "hungry morning" to show up on your food journal. Make a note where you enter your breakfast on your journal if you had one. If not, take a closer look at what you're eating at night.

your spot on the sofa and work on your photos or your closet. Or you might retain your sofa spot but get busy with handy activities that distract you from food. Clients often tell me it feels so weird at first. But you'll soon get used to it, and you'll be surprised to find that the evening can be a great time to get some things accomplished. That positive feeling will reinforce your diet improvements too.

What Late-Night Shufflers Need to Know

USE THE BLUEPRINT TO MANAGE DAYTIME MEALS Some people actually undereat during the day because of all the distractions of their schedule, so that by the time they're home in the evening they truly are starving. The solution: Night eaters *must* eat three real meals a day so hunger is kept under control. And picks and tastes do not count as meals. Here's an essential tip: Because night eaters struggle most with eating after dinner, the most effective strategy is to *delay all meals* a bit if you possibly can so that the third meal—dinner—is later and there is less time between dinner and bedtime. So if you used to have a 7:30 A.M. breakfast, a noon lunch and a 6:00 P.M. dinner, shoot for later times. Your new schedule might be: breakfast at 9:00–9:30, lunch at 1:00–1:30 and dinner at 8:00–8:30. While in general it's better to eat dinner earlier, for Late-Night Shufflers a delayed dinner is more strategic because it cuts out many calories that could otherwise be consumed after dinner and before bed.

GET A JUMP ON HUNGER If you really are starving in the evening, then you need some tips for banishing hunger. Just before dinner, have two glasses of water and an optional plain fiber cracker. This helps take the edge off your hunger and makes you feel a little full. Then add 1–2 cups of extra steamed green veggies like broccoli, string beans or asparagus (no sauce, no salt) to your dinner.

SEAL THE MEAL If you need something sweet after dinner, choose fruit. You must eat it within twenty minutes of dinner. Why? Because you're just trying to enjoy a little sweet and then be done for the night. You don't want to save it for later and turn it into a night-eating habit. Hand fruits, like oranges or bananas are good, as are refreshing slices of grapefruit. You can also try frozen fruit. Seventeen frozen grapes take some time to eat and are delicious. Or you could core and bake an apple—just a few minutes in the micro with a sprinkle of cinnamon if you like—as a delicious treat.

"THE KITCHEN IS CLOSED" I always tell my clients (and remind myself!) that once dinner is over, the kitchen is closed! No wandering in just to take a peek in the fridge during a *Glee* commercial break to see if anything's changed in there. No using the excuse of a few dishes to put in the dishwasher. No. Once you've eaten, you're finished in the kitchen. It's just too hard for Late-Night Shufflers to be in the kitchen without nibbling. If you have a significant other or children, perhaps they could do the afterdinner cleanup. One of my clients told me that she just left the dinner dishes for the next morning. The leftover tidbits stuck to the plates lose a lot of appeal twelve hours later. Just try to get a system down so you can close your kitchen by 9:00 P.M. The only possible reason to enter after that is to perhaps make a cup of herbal tea to enjoy before bed.

THE TURKEY SOLUTION I have had clients who tell me that they just absolutely, positively can't get through the night without a late snack. They're starving beyond description by 11:00 P.M. and they must eat or they can't be responsible for what they might do. Some say they can't sleep if there's nothing in their tummies. For them I devised the Turkey Solution. So if you really *are* hungry, and have to eat, here's the solution: You have two choices: turkey or hard-boiled egg. Pick one. Say you're partial to turkey. Head to the deli and buy a few bags of turkey and ask the counterperson to pack them in ¼-pound bags. When 11:00 P.M. rolls around and you're so hungry you're eyeing the fake fruit on the mantel, take out your bag of turkey and eat it. Most people don't even finish one bag. But if you do finish a whole bag, it's just 150–180 calories. And, by the way, that's simple, straight turkey; no honey turkey or turkey on a cracker or turkey slathered with mustard and pickle. You're not looking for a party; you're looking for a lifeline. If you're more partial to hard-boiled eggs, prepare a few and have them at the ready. Again, if you're starving at near midnight, eat one. Both of these foods will satisfy your hunger without going off the scales, and neither of them will likely set off a binge. They're safe, boring, and healthy and will allow you to sleep while also helping you banish the Late-Night Shuffle.

THE FACE-FREE SOLUTION If you're a vegetarian or you really hate turkey here are two other choices for desperate starvation before bed: any 6–7 ounce yogurt that's 80 calories or less (Greek yogurt is a good choice) or single-serve unsweetened applesauce that's been frozen. Freezing makes it take longer to eat and thus makes it somehow more satisfying. Microwave it for about thirty seconds so it's a little soft and have at it.

DON'T BE FOOLED BY "LITE" SNACKS When I first started working with people who were struggling to lose weight, it was all about calories. Clients would tell me, "Well, I always have evening snacks but it's always low-cal stuff so it's not that bad." Since then we've seen an avalanche of foods that are designed for weight loss, including single-serve treats, low-cal treats and artificially sweetened treats. I learned over time that these treats, especially for Late-Night Shufflers, were a disaster. Sure, they could usually go a night or two having just one low-cal frozen pudding or "healthy" single-serve cupcake. But sure enough, the night would come when they'd lose it and finish the whole box. Remember: Night eating isn't about hunger, it's about habit. The temptation of these so-called healthy foods is that they perpetuate the habit. The real solution is to *break* the habit. That's the only way to free yourself of this dark Devil. So get rid of all the "diet" treats that you may have. If you're really hungry, turn to the Turkey Solution.

FIND A DISTRACTION I mentioned earlier that substituting a good habit for a bad one is the single best way to change your behavior. With that in mind, I suggest that you find some activity to fill your evenings and distract you from the temptations of the fridge. Since stress and anxiety can play a role in night eating, any activity that relieves stress is helpful. I find that accomplishing something at night always calms me and puts me in a positive, powerful mood. There are lots of satisfying little chores that can keep you busy. If you definitely don't want to interfere with your Kardashian habit, give your hands something to do while you're watching. Would knitting or needlework suit you? One client told me she took up knitting and it's been a big help to her. She doesn't want to get the wool dirty with grease from chips or other food stains, so she restricts herself to drinking tea while knitting and catching up on her favorite shows.

You will know what's best for you, but here are some suggestions for evening activities. I suggest you make your own list of the things outside of work that you'd like to accomplish in the evening.

➤ Seasonal organizing: We all seem to be drowning in stuff. Pick a closet, a drawer, a cabinet and thin it out. It is indescribably satisfying to open a drawer and find it neat and organized.

➤ Make an album: Since we all seem to be relying on digital photos these days, it's nice to create an album to print or do something more creative like using your photos to create a storybook to use as a gift or just to have as a keepsake.

➤ Social networking: This can distract you for an entire evening. Just be sure you're not munching as you Facebook or tweet or google your high school sweetheart.

➤ Find a significant other: For singles only, of course. Online dating is a great way to meet new people and expand your social circle. Give it a try. It's better than a bag of popcorn.

➤ Muster an army: You might enjoy zoning out with a flight simulator or some other type of engaging video game. Again, no snacking while playing.

➤ Catch up: Have a friend or relative you haven't spoken with in ages? Always too busy to catch up? After dinner is the perfect time to pick up the phone for a long, satisfying, calorie-free chat.

WATCH WHAT YOU WATCH   Do you find that when you watch TV shows that are all about serial killers, murderous zombies, the end of the world or housewives screaming at one another you begin to feel anxious? Does this anxiety drive you to the fridge? You wouldn't be the first person with this issue. But you may have never before made the connection. So if you find that your shows are prompting anxiety eating, it's time to either change the channel or the activity. Try reading for a change. Maybe an evening spent with your Kindle or iPad or some great magazines would soothe you and also help you avoid the Late-Night Shuffle.

GEOGRAPHIC EATING   Move, move, move . . . away from the kitchen! Do the shut down. If you move out of the living room or kitchen earlier in the night you'll reduce temptation. You have a huge advantage if you live in a two-story house, which gives you the opportunity to move a whole floor away from the fridge. If you close down the house—turn off lights, lock up and move into the bedroom—you'll reinforce the idea that food is over. Even in my tiny apartment with the kitchen right next to the bedroom you'd be amazed at how this technique helps with the temptations of the Late-Night Shuffle. Your geography affects your food choices so make it work for you.

SPA NIGHT   Your dinner is finished and you're settling in for the night. Instead of sinking onto the sofa, do some personal prep work for the morning. Take a shower if you like. Take a lingering bath. Give yourself a manicure or a pedicure; use a face masque. Floss your teeth to a fare-thee-well. Use whitening strips on your teeth (which stop you from eating for at least a half hour!) Most of these personal hygiene activities will help to distract you from the temptation to simply veg out, watch TV and eat, which is the usual routine for night eaters. Moreover, you'll just feel better about yourself as you take control of your time and coddle yourself a bit.

SPOUSE ON A TRIP? Sometimes we can look at our sudden solitude when our partner is out of town as a great opportunity to totally focus on our weight loss goals. How about hunkering down for five nights of frozen dinners and double exercise workouts? Well, the truth is that this plan often backfires. By the third night you're wandering the kitchen, looking for goodies, feeling lonely and figuring out what greasy pile of calories you'll order from the Chinese place. No, no, no. You're not used to being alone and in your heart you're going to feel pathetic and sorry for yourself if you start playing the martyr. A night or two of frozen is good; an obsession with starving yourself alone in your room is bad. Come to the cabaret! Make your own plans. Have a relaxing, healthy dinner with a friend you've not seen in a while. Visit somebody for the evening. Take yourself to a museum and eat in the museum dining room or a nearby casual restaurant alone. Don't punish yourself. You'll feel refreshed and cheerful when your partner returns. And ready to continue working steadily toward your goal.

SINGLE GALS AND GUYS Do you live alone? This can make night eating more of an issue. There's nobody to watch you, nobody to distract you. You might feel lonely . . . a little disconnected. I always advise my single clients to be active outside of work in the evening. It's good for your head and it's the best antidote to the Late-Night Shuffle. Take a class. Almost every neighborhood has learning opportunities that can put you into a new social and intellectual world. It doesn't have to be a class on nuclear disarmament. How about jewelry making? Sculpting? Or the films of Woody Allen? The point is to get out and do something interesting. You'll meet new people and get a real psychological lift. One of my clients took a painting class at night and a few years and many classes later was asked to teach a class at the school she attended, opening up a whole new career for her.

Single people have another great weapon against the Late-Night Shuffle: Exercise! As stress and anxiety play a role in night eating, exercise—a proven stress reducer—is the perfect solution. There are always great exercise classes at night, and you have the freedom to take advantage of them. You might not want to do a heavy cardio routine, but yoga, Pilates, body sculpting and tai chi are terrific stress reducers. Bring along your exercise outfit and you can go right from work to class. Have a super healthy evening: exercise class, home and shower, light frozen dinner, bed! No night eating in that schedule. (Check out "Sloth," page 161 for more specific information on exercise.)

BUST ON OUT   Long evening of munching ahead of you? Time for a change of plan. How about a movie? We all work too hard and get too stressed during the week. We tend to save

Run with a Purpose

Can you picture yourself running a 5K? A 10K? A mini-marathon or even an entire marathon? Most people can't. Until they learn more and join a group that gives instruction and support. There are many organizations out there these days that organize races for fund-raising purposes. You can get training, encouragement and a whole new group of friends, all while getting fit and raising money for a good cause. Team in Training (http://www.teamintraining.org/) is a group that can get you started no matter where you live.

our relaxation for weekends. But sometimes a mid-week movie is just what you need to put some fun in your life (and avoid the Late-Night Shuffle). Have a healthy snack at the end of the day, go enjoy your movie and have one of the frozen dinners when you get home. Then tuck in. Done!

A WARM DRINK IS YOUR LATE-NIGHT FRIEND   Try an herbal tea. It will give your mouth something to do. Chamomile tea is a good nighttime choice. I love the Mighty Leaf Chocolate Mint Truffle Tea. It smells just like a chocolate mint. Celestial Seasonings makes Sleepytime, a flavorful nighttime, caffeine-free tea. Or try a low-cal cocoa: mix 1 teaspoon of Ghiradelli cocoa mix in warm skim milk. It's only about 40 calories and is filling and calming. Swiss Miss has a sugar-free hot chocolate for only 25 calories a serving. Or you can take a cup of unsweetened almond milk (just 40 calories), heat it up and add a dash of cinnamon or nutmeg.

The Late-Night Shuffle Five-Step Cure

If you are a night eater, follow the Blueprint (page 27) carefully. Here's a shorthand version that should help you:

1. Have your dinner at whatever time suits you. But remember that for some people, later is better.

2. Within twenty minutes of dinner, have a piece of fruit if you like. Some people need this bit of dessert; others can skip.

3. After the fruit, if you have it, you're done with food! Now it's liquids only. You can have seltzer, herbal tea or maybe sugar-free hot chocolate. See above for some hot drink suggestions.

4. Do the shutdown as soon as you can: Turn off the lights, lock the door, and move into the bedroom to start winding down.

5. If you're really, truly, madly starving, try the Turkey Solution: Eat a ¼ pound of turkey or a hard-boiled egg.

Do You Use a Sleep Medication?

There are sleep meds that can prompt middle-of-the-night eating. I've had clients who were unaware of this side effect and woke up shocked to find crumbs in the kitchen. If you have this issue, consult your doctor about alternative sleep medications.

Diet Devil #4
Emotional Eating

Most people recognize their Devils fairly easily. But there's one Devil that can lurk quietly and unobtrusively in the background, undermining your best efforts at weight loss. This Devil is Emotional Eating. Almost everyone who has struggled with weight has experienced episodes of Emotional Eating. In fact, it's so common and destructive that I believe it's the major, largely unrecognized, cause of weight gain.

How do you differentiate Emotional Eating from normal, healthy eating? Emotional Eating is eating that's not prompted by hunger or social pressure. Rather it's eating that's prompted by *feelings*: sadness, anger, frustration or stress, to name a few. Complications in relationships with spouses, family, friends, children and coworkers can all cause Emotional Eating. Many of my clients describe Emotional Eating as a sort of out-of-body experience. "I was so angry after the fight with my husband that I finished the whole pint of Ben & Jerry's. I don't think I even tasted it," said one woman. "I was so upset that I then tore into the bag of chips and finished it off." It's distracted, mindless eating and it's utterly unsatisfying. When you're physically hungry, you can delay a meal for a while and make a reasonable choice about what to eat. Emotional Eating, on the other hand, is compulsive and often focused on a particular food (Hello chips! Bring on the ice cream!). Healthy eating makes you feel satisfied; Emotional Eating makes you feel guilty.

Comfort foods are like crack for Emotional Eaters, and carbs are usually their food of choice. Because what's really at the heart of most Emotional Eating is a search for comfort and a longing to be soothed. Unfortunately the price of soothing yourself with a casserole of mac 'n' cheese is high, and failing to recognize Emotional Eating can make reaching your weight loss goals extremely difficult.

Emotional Eaters typically eat when they're sad, depressed, angry, worried, frustrated, ashamed or guilty. But any kind of change can stimulate feelings that prompt Emotional Eating. Divorce, death of a loved one, health issues, a problem with a child, a move, . . . these events throw us off kilter and for many of us the response is to self-medicate with food. I recently had a client who gained over twenty pounds when her husband was diagnosed with a critical illness. Up until his diagnosis, she had always been slim. But it doesn't take a major life change like a life-threatening disease or divorce to prompt Emotional Eating. The stress of raising children, work, financial worries, an argument with a coworker, even holidays or planning a vacation can push us over the edge and into a bag of chips or a big tub of hummus.

Loss of control is this Devil's best friend. Almost any situation that feels out of your control can prompt you to eat. Many of my clients have told me that the very fact of being overweight causes them so much anxiety that they overeat. How frustrating is that? Here's how one of my longtime clients, Suzanne, describes it: "When I first met with Heather and she began to discuss Emotional Eating with me it was all I could do not to cry. I'd been struggling with my weight for a few years and it's almost impossible to describe how depressed it made me. When my clothes were tight or I had to shop for new clothes for

Emotional Shut-Down

Not everyone is plagued by Emotional Eating. Actually the opposite can be true: Some people find that their appetites shut down when their emotions run high. And even for those who *are* Emotional Eaters, not all emotions prompt eating. Interestingly, great excitement or happiness often has the opposite effect. In the first weeks of a romance many people find themselves losing weight. Yet once they're comfortable in a relationship they find that lost weight creeping back. If only we could spend our lives falling in love.

an occasion, I got so upset that I'd wind up just having some ice cream or pizza. It was almost as if I ate so I wouldn't cry. But once I could step back and recognize how emotions were making me eat, the picture in my head changed and I regained some control. Just naming this issue—Emotional Eating—made a huge difference. Finally I could tell myself that I wasn't hungry and didn't want to eat and that I was just feeling bad or anxious about something. Only then did I begin to lose."

You do not have to be victimized by Emotional Eating. The key words here are *recognition* and *control*. I'm going to help you recognize what's going on in your mind that's making you eat more than you want. We'll take a look at some issues that plague Emotional Eaters. And then I'm going to give you some foolproof strategies that will help you gain control of your situation so the pounds will begin to disappear.

What Emotional Eaters Need to Know

THE EMOTIONAL EATER'S FOOD JOURNAL Earlier in the book, I discussed the importance of keeping a food diary. This applies especially to Emotional Eaters. If you haven't completed a few weeks of your food journal, now's the time to work on it. (See "FreeStyle Dieting," page 83.) Follow the suggestions there: Write down everything you eat and the time of day. In addition, you should add two notes to your journal:

➤ Make sure you make a note of how you're feeling when you eat. Were you angry when you had that snack? Depressed at dinner? Lonely at bedtime? Here's a list of emotions you might want to refer to throughout your week when identifying feelings that make you eat:

Sad	Frustrated	Guilty
Lonely	Angry	Ashamed
Fearful	Stressed	

Scan through your journal to determine if there's a connection between negative feelings and overeating. If you're an Emotional Eater you'll probably discover that your moods have a big effect on what and how much you eat.

➤ Don't forget to note the Triumphs in your food journal. Emotional Eaters sometimes find it too easy to denigrate themselves. So pause and record anything you've done that's been a positive step forward to your weight goal. This might be walking to the store instead of driving; passing up on the breadbasket while out to dinner or reaching your daily water goal. Give yourself a break and a pat on the back.

TAKE A STEP BACK What's stressing you? What are you anxious about? Sometimes there's nothing you can actually *do* about a stress but simply by recognizing it you'll reduce the pressure. Take a minute right now and make a quick list of the things that are stressing you. One client came to me after she started a new job and within four months gained fifteen pounds. She couldn't figure out why this was happening, and her weight gain was making her feel more and more anxious and helpless. In the course of our conversation it quickly became apparent that she was an Emotional Eater who was overwhelmed by the demands of her new boss. She was snacking constantly and just couldn't find a way to stop. She told me that her "willpower had evaporated."

The first thing I helped her understand was that she wasn't suffering from a failure of "willpower" but rather from unremitting stress that made her turn to food for distraction and comfort. It was a tremendous help for her to make the connection between her anxiety about her new position and her eating. She had come to feel that her life was completely out of control. By our second session she was taking active measures to change her eating habits and soon felt calmer and more positive. While she couldn't control her boss, she *could* control her reaction to her situation and her food intake. As she began to lose weight she also began to think about switching to another position within the same company that would be less stressful. She told me at our third session that she'd made the job move and now could remind herself, "You don't want to eat; you want to relax." This helped her to redirect her energies and avoid the snacking that had been tempting her.

Whether or not you can change the sources of stress in your life, it's important to keep in mind that the one thing you *always* have control over is what you eat. This should be your mantra when it comes to Emotional Eating: I can't control everything in my life, but I can control what I put in my mouth.

SET A GOAL AND REACH IT Nothing makes you feel more in control than reaching a goal, even if it's a simple one. I suggest that clients start each day with one or two—you might even jot them down in your food journal. It may be food related, such as, "Today I'm going to have my healthy snack at 4:00 P.M. and then nothing until dinner." Or maybe it's work related, like, "Today I'm going to spend an hour working on that report that's due on Friday." Or it could be a family goal: "Today I'll spend an hour with my toddler at the park." Plan to succeed. When you do, you'll boost your sense of confidence and you'll find that everything in your life will seem more achievable.

EMBRACE STRESS MANAGEMENT   If your Emotional Eating is largely due to stress—and for many people, that's the root cause—there are techniques to get your stress under control. Meditation is an extremely effective way of releasing stress. It's also a terrific deterrent to Emotional Eating. When you feel an urge to overeat, take five minutes, close your eyes and concentrate on your breathing. Get a kitchen timer to keep track of the time so you can keep your eyes closed and focus entirely on breathing deeply. Research has shown that meditation, practiced regularly, can actually change your brain. I know for sure that it can divert an impulse to eat and help strengthen your resolve. Yoga can also help with stress control, and these days it's pretty easy to find a yoga class that suits you.

LEARN TO RECOGNIZE PHYSICAL HUNGER   Many of my clients who are Emotional Eaters have become totally disconnected from the feeling of physical hunger. They eat when they think they're supposed to eat—breakfast, lunch, dinner—but then they snack compulsively and mindlessly when they're feeding a feeling: after a difficult meeting, when they're worried about a family member or any number of similar situations. If this is true for you, connect with your physical hunger by noting in your food diary how hungry you are each time *before* you eat, ranking it from 1 (not hungry) to 10 (absolutely starving). There's no point in having a snack if you're not really hungry. In fact, you may sometimes not be very hungry at mealtime. If this is the case, don't skip a meal but, rather, eat lightly. If you don't want a big breakfast, have some yogurt and fruit. Or perhaps a salad and grilled chicken or fish will satisfy you at dinner. Try one of the very low-cal frozen dinners. Once you're in touch with your hunger, you're in the driver's seat.

FIND ANOTHER COMFORT   You know that anxious, fidgety feeling that makes you want to open up a sleeve of crackers and just down them, one after the other? There's no denying that eating can be comforting. Carbs in particular are soothing. When you endure chronic stress, your brain cells are bathed in the hormone cortisol, which makes you crave fatty, salty, sweet, crunchy foods. Those carbs that you then crave temporarily calm you. But the good feeling wears off very quickly and soon you're back to craving more. And feeling bad about what you've already consumed. Thus the vicious cycle of Emotional Eating. An excellent and very effective strategy is to find something to do that will distract you both from your stress and from the elusive comfort of food. Some of these sound obvious but if you make a short list of a few that appeal to you, you'll find that when cravings strike you'll be prepared to direct your attention elsewhere.

ARE THINGS REALLY OUT OF YOUR CONTROL?   Emotional Eaters tend to believe that they just have to live with whatever is stressing them and prompting them to eat. Some people even believe that eating is the only way they have to deal with their problems. So let's pause for a moment and take a look at what's out of kilter in your life. I'm not a therapist, but I do know from long experience that when people feel victimized by situations they often turn to food. But once you take a clear look at what's prompting you to overeat you may be able to

"Cut Your Hair" Friends!

Not everyone is thrilled to see you losing weight and looking good. Don't you have at least a couple of frenemies who would enjoy meowing at your muffin top? I call them "cut your hair" friends. "Yes, you would definitely look good with a super-short pixie!" It's not only their beauty advice that can trip you up: They can be dedicated pie pushers! Because if you are out of control, they feel better by comparison. Yes, it's sad. But if you're not alert to these folks you could wind up pounds heavier. Try to avoid eating out with them if you can. Never stand next to them in a buffet line. And if they present you with chocolates or cupcakes, have a plan. The best way to cope with "cut your hair" friends is to simply be alert to their nefarious ways. Then you can be prepared to stick to your resolutions with a smile and leave them in the mean girl dust. Stealth Dieting is really your baseline defense against "cut your hair" friends. Read all about it in "Dine Out Devils" (page 217).

change your situation or at least recognize it for what it is and not allow it to stand in the way of your goal to eat healthfully. I often say to clients, "Would you rather be thin and stressed/anxious/frustrated or heavy and stressed/anxious/unhappy?" We all know the answer to that, and sometimes it's empowering to make a decision not to let emotional issues interfere with your healthy plans.

THE FAT KID HANGOVER　Were you heavy as a child? Some people who were fat as children become super determined to lose weight and never let it creep up again. And they're strong and successful at it. Other people face a constant struggle. There can be so much baggage involved. People who never resolved their childhood struggles can be very sensitive about weight and can easily get sent down the path to overeating.

Sometimes parents are part of the problem, and this makes the situation doubly complicated. I've certainly seen the difficulties that people have over this. The best advice I can give is to try to let the issue go. Make a choice to move on and check it off your list. Food is always going to be a part of our lives, and it's worth the struggle to make peace with it. If you can't lose weight and you think your childhood issues have something to do with it, you could benefit from some counseling that will help you recognize your complicated feelings and resolve them.

MAN, OH MANOREXIC   Are you living with a guy who has become obsessed with what he eats? Maybe he's had a pep talk or scare talk from his doctor and has totally cleaned up his eating act. Maybe he's become a gym rat who thinks of nothing but his abs. It's very stressful to have a partner (male or female, for that matter) who's turned into a Dining Devil. It can be especially challenging when the Devil is male. Men tend to have no inhibitions about sharing their obsessions with all and sundry. They can sit at dinner with a handful of overweight people and proudly discuss their lack of body fat while their companions want to sob into their napkins. They can tell your best friend that she shouldn't be eating that apple because it has fructose in it. (Wha??) And, of course, they can be telling you exactly what to eat and when if you want to be buff and beautiful just like them. It's enough to send you right to the Milk Duds, if not to couples' therapy. No one likes to have eating turn into a competition, nor to be told what to eat. And of course it's a stereotype but women tend to like a guy "who eats." It can be irritating to have a guy order a perfect dinner or tell the waiter to "hold the fries; they're fattening."

How do you handle this? First, you simply have to recognize it's happening. Understand that it can be a good thing that your partner is health conscious. Don't let it push you into poor choices just to retaliate—an understandable reaction but, face it, crazy! And here's what I've learned about men and food. Many men do not have the complicated relationship with food that women do. So when they discover healthy eating, they want to tell the world. It's your job to have a talk with him and tell him that it's not appropriate to bang the drum for celery in public. Put a sock in it. It's great that he's taking care of his health; it's not great that he's driving people, including you, away. Teach him how to be a Stealth Dieter. (Show him how to make Stealth Orders in restaurants [page 217].) And try to work it out so you're not competing on the Amazing Food Race but rather so that you're a *team* of healthy eaters.

DATE EATING   Remember what it was like when you went on those first dates with someone you were really excited about? You had no appetite, right? No interest in food. Mallomars, who cares? I've had clients who struggled with their scale and then met someone special and suddenly the pounds melted away. But of course all good things come to an end. You get engaged. You get married. Or you just move in together. The boiling excitement simmers down and you're comfortable. Courting is over and here come the happy pounds. This happens in part because most men can eat more than women and once you're living together you boost your intake to match his. There's also the undeniable fact that coupleship can sometimes cause stress that can prompt you to eat. If you're in a new relationship, enjoy the melting pounds phenomena. If you're starting to settle in with someone, don't let your partner's higher calorie intake sweep you along. It's really a matter of paying attention. Following my Blueprint will help you stay focused on staying slim. And keep the conversation going: Talk to your partner about how important it is for you to stay healthy and look good. Eating well is the cornerstone of that goal.

First Date Tip

Many of my clients are young singles, looking for romance. Of course they're seeing me because they're struggling with their weight. And sometimes they become so immersed in the world of carbs and fiber that they lose perspective. So I tell all my lady clients to take a step back: When you're on a first date, relax! Share the dessert. Eat the hot dog at the game. Don't be high maintenance. He doesn't really care about your diet. You've got to be cool in the beginning of a relationship. Once he says he loves you, you can pull out your lean order. But no special requests on the first date. You'll lose weight out of happiness anyhow. (See "Stealth Dieting," page 217, for tips on how to trick your date into thinking you're a carefree eater.)

RELATIONSHIP EATING   Yes, more on relationships . . . important people in our lives can really affect our eating habits, positively or negatively. One can eat a lot; the other can't. One couldn't care less about healthy eating; the other is concerned.

The biggest complaint I hear from men about the women in their lives centers on "picking." As one guy said, "Weekends drive me crazy. She eats constantly but she never really finishes anything. She's always snacking but never really eating."

Many women have a similar complaint: He eats constantly. Most men do finish the food. But they don't finish cleaning up after the food! And they eat tempting things that draw their lady pals into treats that they'd rather avoid.

If you're living in a situation where you and your partner have very different eating styles, you have to keep the conversation going. You have to work it out. I always say, "Have the conversation, not the fight." Make your partner part of your team. Maybe you need to rely on frozen dinners once or twice a week when your partner just must have a steak. We do surf and turf at our house: My husband loves a steak and I love fish. While he's grilling a steak, I'm popping my fish into the toaster oven. Maybe you need to teach yourself to pour a tonic or seltzer when your partner is on that third glass of wine with dinner. In my house, we have the peanut butter wars. I can't rest when there's peanut butter in the pantry. My husband refused to believe that a nutritionist couldn't control herself around a small plastic jar. Many empty jars of peanut butter later I got him to agree to a truce: If he must have peanut butter in the house, then he must hide it. Every so often, I find it. And then he finds a new hiding place. No more fights. No more (or many fewer) peanut butter binges for me. That's the key: Adaptation. You may change some things about your partner, but you're probably not going to change the way he or she eats. But that's no reason to abandon your healthy goals. Just keep the conversation going and focus on working it out.

MOMMY DEAREST   What could be more complicated than a mother-daughter relationship? You arrive back home, mom opens the front door and there's that pause when she looks you up and down. . . . There's boundless love and a powerful connection. But there can also be underlying jealousy and competition. This can be expressed through food and weight. If mom is petite and daughter is not, it can cause a big issue between them. I've had clients who tell me that their moms are constantly asking them if they've lost any weight. This can be infuriating and can drive you right into the fridge. (There's nothing like being told what to eat or not eat to make you want to do the opposite!) Again, I'm not a therapist. Only you know if you can discuss your feelings with your mom and if that discussion would be beneficial. But if your mom makes you feel uncomfortable about your weight, it could be worth trying to explain your feelings to her. At the very least, recognize what is happening with your mom and don't let your negative feelings prompt you to lose control.

TAKE ADVANTAGE OF "SET YOUR CLOCK" FRIENDS   I have a friend, Kate, who started out as my running buddy but evolved into what I call my "set your clock" friend. When I want a night out where I know I'm going to be able to have a perfectly clean dinner, plus have fun and get a "health boost," Kate's the one I call. We go out and have some grilled fish, a salad, lots of water, maybe one glass of wine and lots of fun conversation. I go home, brush my teeth, text Kate that I'm not having any treats at home and I wake up feeling great the next day. A "set your clock" friend is someone to encourage you, support you and make clean eating fun. So grab your sister, your cousin, your best friend. They'll pick you up when you're down and make losing more fun.

DRESS FOR DIET SUCCESS   How you look has a significant effect on how you feel. When you're having a great hair day, wearing your slimming power suit and your sexy heels or your slim jeans and your super-flattering sweater, you feel on top of the world, in control and ready to take on anything. And when you're sporting your sloppy sweats and your hair is fried, the last thing you feel able to do is face and conquer the world. You don't even want to answer the door! If you're an Emotional Eater one of your goals—and you really should actively focus on this—is to make yourself feel great, and a short cut to that goal is a great outfit. Spend some time on your appearance. Most of my clients who are overweight when they first come to see me resist this message. But I insist that they find at least one outfit for home or work that looks really terrific on them and wear it regularly. In addition, I ask them—and you—to ditch the baggy clothes. You don't have to wear a leotard but I promise you that loose-fitting clothes are a major deterrent to weight loss. When you can feel your waistband you are less inclined to binge. It's just too uncomfortable.

AVOID THE CANCELS Have you ever noticed that when you're feeling in a funk or you've been eating badly you're tempted to cancel plans? You'd so much rather hide under the covers than have to get dressed in clothes that feel tight, and you're in such bad spirits that you don't feel like you have anything to contribute to any gathering. Plus you may convince yourself that you'll be tempted to eat unhealthy food and then you'll feel even worse and further out of control. Years ago my husband told me that friends were calling us "the Cancels" instead of the Bauers. This forced me to think about why I was opting out of so many invitations. In part I was canceling because I really am more of a homebody. But I can't deny that I was also canceling because I didn't want to squeeze into a tight pair of jeans and go out and eat unhealthy foods. But this avoidance strategy was really backfiring on me since I found when I stayed home I felt so guilty that I'd sink into a mishmash dinner and consume more calories than if I'd gone out. It's important to be social. You'll see a friend or maybe meet someone special if you're single and you'll have networking opportunities. If you don't feel at your best physically, work it: Get a blow out or a manicure or some new shoes. No one will notice your weight if you dress in black and wear something flattering. If your jeans are tight, wear something looser; your clothes will soon be loose as you work on your clean eating. And that's another reason to go out: Evening plans can help you stay on track during the day. Think of it as "date day eating": super-clean meals so you can feel your best for the evening activities. And if someone cancels on you? Don't let yourself feel bad. See it as an opportunity to have a clean night with a frozen dinner and some personal pampering.

SNOOZE TO LOSE Are you running ragged? Stretched as tight as your Spanks? Limping along on five or six hours of

sleep per night? Did it ever occur to you that sleep deprivation can boost your appetite? Oh yes. Researchers tell us that
lack of sleep can wreak havoc on the hormones that control
your appetite. Too little sleep means too much appetite. You
might have noticed this. You wake up exhausted after a few
hours sleep and the only thing you can think of that might
make you feel better is something loaded with carbs and calories. How about a giant stack of pancakes swimming in syrup
and butter? Oh yes; that will perk me up. Oh no it won't! If
you want to reduce the struggle you sometimes have with
your appetite, give it every advantage; get a good night's
sleep. Turn off your favorite evening talk shows. Develop a
healthy nighttime routine. Most people require at least seven
to eight hours of sleep every night. If you're getting less than
this on a regular basis, you could be sabotaging your efforts
to lose weight.

EXERCISE   Sloth is a Diet Devil that I describe more fully on
page 161, but lack of exercise can contribute to Emotional Eating. I'll just mention here that if you are a total couch potato
you are more likely to fall victim to Emotional Eating. Exercising makes you feel in control. It boosts endorphins and
mood. You don't have to be a marathoner to benefit from
exercise—just take a walk around the block or take the dog for
a walk or toss a ball with your child next time you feel the
urge to snack. Your blood will start flowing and you may well
forget all about your urge to nibble.

FAMILY MAKEOVER   It can be challenging to eat clean and
healthy if you are surrounded by junk food junkies. If your
family regularly eats tubs of fried foods, bins of chips and vats
of soda, it may be time to do a whole family food intervention
and reconsider the foods you have around the house and what

> ## Find a Text Buddy
>
> Have a friend who's trying to lose weight too? Make a pact: Text your food intake to one another. It's like a living food journal with some emotional support. It can keep you honest and make it fun. Of course you need to have a very supportive and honest friend. But try it. It can be a great way to stay on track.

your family, particularly your children, eat. There are so many healthy cookbooks and online sites that will give you great ideas. Enlist your family in making healthy changes. Even the youngest children can learn to help in the kitchen and that fellow with the chicken parm sauce on his chin can probably find his way around the perimeter of the supermarket if asked.

If you find that your family's eating style is a real deterrent to your weight loss efforts, it might be time to simply enlist their help. Sit them down and have a talk with them. Tell them how you feel about trying to eat healthy food and how they can help you—and how you *need* their help to stay on track. When the family sees how much it means to you to reach your new goals, they surely will become your biggest allies and healthy eating will become a family affair.

GET SOME OUTSIDE SUPPORT You can't always handle everything by yourself. Sometimes you need some help. If you are feeling really stressed about something and just can't see a way out, it may be time to get some assistance from a mental health professional. Perhaps a therapist would give you the perspective that will get you through difficult times. Perhaps a support group of some kind could be the answer. Every now and again I've had clients whose Emotional Eating was prompted by something so overwhelming that they needed more than dieting strategies to see their way clear. If you think that describes your situation, take a look at what resources your community might have to help get you over this rough patch in your life.

Diet Devil #5
Little Devils

Oh yes, the joy of your life . . . your children. They complete you. They give your life meaning. They fill your days with . . . food! That's right. While your children may well be the best thing that ever happened to you, they are probably not the best things that ever happened to your waistline. Indeed, they make you gain weight before you even lay eyes on them. Children and food: Can't have one without the other.

A Note for Dad

Even though you are not growing a baby in your belly, Dad, you shouldn't skip to the next section. Not only will you learn a lot about what your wife is dealing with, you will also learn some perhaps surprising tips about how to avoid the poundage creep that can accompany parenthood. Did you know that the average dad gains fourteen pounds in the course of his partner's pregnancy? In one British study not only did the average dad pack on those extra pounds, he also added about two inches to his waistline. And of course Dad's sympathetic pregnancy doesn't disappear when the baby arrives!

Before you even get the exciting news about the new addition, the stress of getting pregnant can put many women (and their husbands) over the edge in terms of food consumption. The decision to get pregnant isn't always a simple one, and it can prompt an eating festival that we justify with the excuse that we're trying to eat healthy foods . . . lots of them. Sometimes there's the disappointment if a pregnancy doesn't succeed. And what about the stress that's inevitable when one partner is more excited about growing the family than the other? And for those who have to endure fertility treatments, there's another source of stress—and stress eating—as well as the additional pounds that can come along with the hormones involved in treatments.

Once you're pregnant, weight gain can become a major preoccupation. For some of us, pregnancy is the first step in a long-term struggle with weight. This isn't surprising. For one thing, you're eating for two! Hooray, right? Well, not so fast: The fact is that you only need an average of 300 extra calories daily to grow a baby, and that amounts to a decaf venti soy latte and a big banana. Nonetheless, many women see pregnancy as a license to pack on the pounds, figuring that they'll all evaporate with childbirth. There are a number of reasons for this abandonment of reason. For one thing, your usual measures of weight gain are no longer reliable. Your pants are tight? Of course they are! You can't button your blouse? No surprise there. All the boundaries that have helped keep you in check have evaporated, or, rather, expanded.

In addition to losing your usual boundaries, you might become preoccupied with food. You may be nauseated in the early months, and for many women this becomes a license to chow down big time when the nausea passes.

At last baby arrives and you begin to adjust to a new life as a family. Some moms want to just settle in for the first few weeks; others are eager to work on getting back to their

How Much You Can Expect to Lose with Childbirth

Most women lose only about twelve pounds. Of course, your body retained lots of fluid to sustain your pregnancy, and most new moms notice that they produce more urine immediately after birth—up to an amazing 3 quarts a day for many women. And then there's the sweating! Most women lose roughly an additional four pounds of water weight by the time their baby is a week old. Of course your results may vary: I returned from the hospital after birthing my 7.5-pound daughter weighing exactly what I weighed going in!

prepregnancy weight immediately. (I have had clients text me from the hospital for tips on regaining their prepregnancy shape.) Either approach is fine. The first step in taking off the baby weight is to focus on good, healthy eating. For one thing, moms who eat well and as regularly as they can will simply be more energetic and healthy and better able to care for baby. And it's never too early to start being a good example to your little one.

Once your baby has settled into a routine you'll begin to confront the issues that Little Devils create in your life that can confound even the most determined mom. Why? Fatigue is a huge issue. When you're tired, you want to eat. And what do you reach for? Those Devil Carbs! Lack of time is another huge issue for new moms. Whether or not you're working outside the home, a baby absorbs a tremendous amount of time. This may be time that you used to spend on shopping for and cooking healthy meals or on exercising. As a mother of three, including a set of twins, I know all about the time crunch that every parent experiences, and I'll give you some tips below on how you can manage your weight while still raising your children. If you're a working mom you're probably going to face another issue: the stress of always wanting to be in two places at once! It's tough for working moms, especially when their kids are small. No matter how much you love your job, there are going to be times when all you want is to be with your children. This stress can prompt anxious eating.

And what about that plump fellow sitting on the sofa with a diaper on his shoulder? Dad's not exempt from baby blubber. After all, he's living right in the center of stress central, too, not to mention the fatigue. He's listening to the crying. He's probably getting up at night. And he's suddenly, if it's a first child, trying to figure out how to grow up and be a dad ASAP. The simple truth is that it's a huge adjustment: Who's going to pick up the baby? Why isn't dad as "bonded" as mom? How are the in-laws dealing with all this? Talk about stressful! And that leads to food and weight gain.

On the very bright side being a parent is the best motivation ever for losing weight and getting into the best shape of your life. You have the most important reason you'll ever have to be

Your Children and Food Issues

I know you're concerned with weight and losing it, and you may have had years of struggles with food. But it's important to remember that you want your children to have healthy attitudes toward food and the best way to give them that gift is to be a good example. Your children look to you as a role model and until about the age of seven or so they want nothing more than to be just like you. So it's important to be positive about food and eating. Get them excited about cooking and trying different foods. Remember that just because you don't like asparagus, there's no reason why your child might not love it. Sometimes it takes a dozen tries before your baby will eat a food; keep trying because on that thirteenth try he may gobble it up.

healthy and energetic and an example of how to live life to the fullest. So let's get started!

Need to Knows for Little Devils

TAKE A FOUR-WEEK PASS   If you are eager to get started on weight control immediately, that's fine. But if you don't feel motivated, give yourself a break. Let the first four weeks ride. Don't focus on your weight while your baby is settling into a routine. You will lose those pounds! The first twenty pounds will come off in time with little effort. But right now you have to adjust to your new role as a mom and enjoy that wonderful baby.

HEALTHY RESTART   You'd have to live under a rock not to know that we are all facing a major obesity epidemic. Our kids are just as vulnerable as we are. Maybe more so because they're going to be exposed to lots of fast food, salty snacks and oceans of soda before they fly the nest. It's your job to encourage a healthy attitude toward food. In my opinion, that means mainly setting a good example. Adding a new baby to your life is the perfect occasion to revise your own nutritional life. A great beginning is to clean up your kitchen. Toss all the un-healthy treats and snacks. Cross soda off your shopping list for good. Don't be lured into buying giant bins of sweet or salty treats at warehouses. You'll be doing your kids a huge favor if you get them off on the right nutritional track with healthy snacks of fruits and vegetables and treats like homemade pop-corn. If your kids don't start out with unhealthy foods, they won't expect them. I'm not suggesting that you ban all sweets. I know that wouldn't work in my house and it probably wouldn't work in yours. But it's wonderful to grow up in a household that embraces healthy food but doesn't obsess about unhealthy food. With some effort on your part, your child can grow up devil-free!

TWO HOURS A WEEK I always tell my moms to try to give themselves two hours every week for food planning and prep time. You can do it on Saturday or Sunday when your partner can take over or while the kids are napping or while you're watching soccer practice from the sidelines. Take this time to map out your week: dinners at home, dinners out, shopping list, and so on. Food stores that deliver are a fantastic help. I'm in New York, where food delivery is easy to arrange, and I make my order on Saturday for a Sunday delivery. Then on Sunday night I can do my prep: Hard-boil some eggs, wash the greens, wash and slice the peppers, cucumbers, celery and store them in Tupperware. I've got my Greek yogurt, Kashi Go Lean cereal, apples, berries, ¼ pound bags of low-sodium organic turkey, my frozen spinach or broccoli and frozen organic meals. This sets me up for a week of easy, quick meals. Your list will depend on your week's activities and your family preferences. The key words are *planning* and *organizing*! And just two hours a week can do it.

STOP PICKING It's so tempting. That mouthful of mac 'n' cheese on the highchair tray. Those crusts from the PB&J. The bubble of pudding in the bottom of the cup. Don't do it! Those bits and smidges can add up to plenty of calories. Even that piece of broccoli, which seems so innocent and low-cal, can encourage the habit of mindless picking. Moreover they can lead you to a Plunge (see page 87) in which you'll find yourself scouring the back of the pantry for forgotten bags of chocolate chips. And even if they're grey and hard, you'll eat them! But no kidding, it's hard to feed children and not follow your natural Mrs. Clean impulse to Hoover up the crumbs. A good way to avoid picking off their plates is to eat with your children when you can. You won't be picking if your own food is in front or you. Some people manage to have breakfast and dinner with the kids; others just breakfast. Whatever you can manage, it's good for your waistline and good for the kids to see mom and dad eating healthy meals.

Other surefire techniques for beating this Devil?

➤ Pop a breath strip in your mouth.

➤ Rely on your bottle of water.

➤ Try chewing sugarless gum.

One strategy that works for me is to have my own cut-up cucumbers or peppers in front of me while my kids eat. (In the past, I would sometimes have an energy bar, but my daughter would beg for a bite so I gave that up.) I nibble on those veggies and if the kids beg for a piece, great!

AVOID DOUBLE DINNERS   Your child needs to eat dinner at say, 5:00 or 6:00 P.M. But your spouse doesn't get home from work until 7:30 or 8:00 P.M. and can't eat until then. What to do? Unless you plan for this you'll find yourself eating double dinners most nights. I struggle with this dilemma in my own household. I tell my clients to simply make a decision: Pick an early or a late dinner and eat only at that time. For example, I know that if I eat with my kids and then sit down to socialize with my husband at his later dinner, I'm going to be picking off his plate or else just serving myself another whole dinner. So I plan to eat my full dinner with my husband. If you plan to have a late dinner with your spouse, it can work well to save your afternoon snack to enjoy while your kids are eating their dinner. Have cut-up cucumber or peppers. I sometimes sip chai tea while feeding my kids.

MANAGE WEEKENDS   Weekends are a whole different experience when you're a family instead of a couple. You may be spending a lot more time around the house (i.e., kitchen), particularly when your kids are young. Your meal schedule may be skewed. You need to focus on managing your time and your food intake. For my best tips on how to handle weekends, see Boredom Bingeing (page 145). But in a nutshell, if you want to get through a clean weekend, start strong: Have a healthy dinner on Friday night and not a pizza binge. And commit to a clean breakfast on Saturday: Don't fall into the pancake trap, or you'll be vulnerable to a totally lost weekend. One tip that most people find extremely effective for those days when they're wandering the house, munching, munching, munching, is to set a start time. The late afternoon is a common time to begin feeling that weird combination of hungry and bored. So make a decision that, for example, you're not going to eat anything at all for the next hour, or hour and a half. If it's 3:30, you're going to eat nothing until 4:30 or 5:00 (assuming your dinner won't be until 7:00 or so). Then allow yourself a healthy snack. You'll see how just setting up these rules in your head makes it easier to stay strong. And don't forget, water, water, water!

AVOID STEALTH (TROJAN HORSE) GOODIE PURCHASES   You know you've done it: bought your favorite treat "for the kids." I used to wander through Whole Foods and toss a bag of organic cheddar bunnies into my cart. I'd stuff it in the pantry and then, at some point when I was really hungry, I'd open it and serve my daughter a small bowl. . . . Which she would ignore because she isn't interested in that type of snack. So I'd eat them. One bowl, two bowl, red bowl, blue bowl. Many of my clients have this bad habit. This is something you have to stop.

MANAGE MONSTER MOMS   Be wary of these moms. They're the ones who make snide comments like, "Wow, your little Susie sure packed on the pounds this summer." Or "Oh, you must be sooo sad that tomorrow's Monday and you have to work and leave your kids." Or, the ever-popular, "You must be so nervous about Tommy's school application. I was a wreck until Joe got in." It's amazing how competitive some mothers can be. What does this have to do with your weight loss? Sometimes these people can make you feel so bad that you bury yourself in a bag of chips. Or, worse, you begin to question your child's weight and your own approach to healthy eating. Best way to repel these cootie moms: Eat clean and strong! When you're in control, you develop an invisible shield, which protects you from monster moms and repels their slings and arrows.

DINING WITH DAUGHTERS   Do you have boys or girls or both? It *does* make a difference. This may sound like a gross generalization but it's true: When it comes to food, boys are easy. Most of them are like farm animals: You just pitchfork it to them and it disappears. Some eat a little; some eat a lot, but few of them have any questions about the process. Girls are another story. They pay attention to food and they're very aware of what you're eating and what you're feeding them and why. It's important to emphasize eating for health with your daughter as opposed to "getting skinny." We all know that there's too much emphasis on being model thin in our culture and that this can cause all manner of grief to young girls. The most important antidote to this skewed emphasis is *you*. Your daughter is watching you all the time. If she's overhearing you comment on "your fat jeans" or how you can't eat this or that because you're dieting, she's going to begin to see food as the enemy.

SNACK TIME   Every kid and every household is different. If I have one message in this book it's that we're all different and you have to know yourself and your children. That holds true when it comes to snacks. Some families can have treat or snack drawers of food and that works for them. If we did that in my house, we'd be eating treats day and night. So I only get healthy snacks in portion-controlled servings like string cheese, yogurt, and cottage cheese or fresh-cut fruit and veggies. That being said, I think it's important to keep watch over even "healthy" snacks. In excess, they're no longer healthy. And they can spoil your child's appetite for wholesome meals. A bigger problem that snacks can pose is that they lead you into temptation. It's tough to hand out crackers or bunches of grapes or slices of apple without nibbling. In fact, if you're someone who needs snacks (read more about this in the Blueprint), you might plan to have your snack with your child. If handing out kiddie snacks is too tempting for you, the breath strip strategy that I mentioned earlier can help. It's not too hard to pass on a handful of crackers when you've got the taste of mint in your mouth. Remember, you can always have turkey, cut-up cucumbers, peppers, celery or a piece of fruit. You're never going to want to binge on these.

THE HOME-ALL-DAY HUNGRIES   It's a joy to spend quality time with your child, but it can also be very isolating. And, let's be honest, boring. I spend some days at my office and some days at home and for me it's definitely harder to eat well at home. If you're a stay-at-home mom, it's sometimes hard to avoid mindless nibbling. After all, you spend quite a bit of time in the kitchen, and it's hard to pretend that it's not full of food. This situation can be especially challenging if you used to work outside the home and therefore had lots of structure and distraction in your day. Check out the tips for Boredom Bingers (page 145) for ways to handle the temptation to make every minute an occasion for a snack. The most important advice I have for stay-at-home parents is to try to create as much of a schedule in your day as possible. Structure is your friend when it comes to weight loss. No matter if you have an infant who's nursing every three hours or a three-year-old who seems to want to nibble constantly, try to eat *your* meals at regular times.

AVOID FOOD REWARDS If you're a working parent it's oh so easy to become the treatmaster. You feel guilty for working and not spending every moment with your child, so the first thing you want to do when you come in the door after work is coax a big smile out of your child with a cupcake or a secret stash of soda or maybe a special cookie. And of course if he or she doesn't finish it or doesn't want it, you get the double pleasure of being the hero and eating the treat. This is bad for everyone. The child quickly figures out that treats are some kind of currency, best enjoyed in a little cloud of guilt, and you introduce an unhealthy eating pattern for both you and your child. If you don't have those secret treats around, you can't rely on them. And the truth is that what your child would like best is a few minutes of your undivided attention, not a cupcake. A game of peek-a-boo or reading a book together is calorie free and ultimately more satisfying than any food treat.

MANAGE BIRTHDAY PARTIES Childhood is a festival. And it should be. Birthdays, Halloween, Christmas, snow days—and they all seem to focus on food. It's great to enjoy cake at a birthday party or a handful of candy on Halloween or some Christmas cookies that Grandma made, but it's not okay for your child or *you* to hoard the three bags of Halloween candy and nibble daily until Thanksgiving! Try to make the focus of holidays more than food and try to make holiday food reasonably healthy. Of course you want to enjoy your family's traditional foods but these days there are countless ways to slim down that green bean–cream cheese–fried onion ring casserole.

Another tip: Put a time limit on holidays. I had a client who told me that Halloween began on October 1 for her family when she went to the big box store and bought drums of candy.

She'd eaten so many mini Butterfingers that by Halloween she could barely stand to answer the door for trick-or-treaters. I broke the news to her that stores are open on Halloween and she could buy her candy that afternoon so its shelf life in her household could be only twenty-four hours!

How do you handle birthday parties? Kids' birthday parties usually mean something to nibble on for the parents and then pizza and cake for everyone. If it's your child's party, you need to be flexible: Have some pizza; have some cake. Call it two carbs and make sure your next meal is a healthy one. If you find that you're attending two or three birthday parties a month, it's time to make a rule: My advice is to skip the cake and go with the pizza. (Pick plain cheese pizza if you have a choice.) Call that one slice your lunch or your dinner. Some clients ask if they can skip the pizza and go for the cake. I think that's a bad idea. Most of the people who ask this are the ones who will have the cake and then slide into a devastating Plunge. So enjoy your one slice of pizza and be done with it. If you know that there's no way you can control yourself with pizza or cake, have a meal before the party so that you're full when you get there and spend your time blowing up balloons, drinking water and breaking up fights.

FINESSE FAST FOOD   Most children are exposed to their first McDonald's french fry before they can even walk. It's very hard to avoid. Indeed, it's not long before the press of soccer practice, homework, play dates and road trips makes the lure of fast food irresistible. Of course you'll want to minimize your child's and your own exposure to the dinner in a bag, but it's good to know that there really are some tasty, healthy choices to be found at fast-food chains all across the country. You can always pick a chicken Caesar salad with balsamic dressing at McDonald's. Your kids will be more interested in the toy in the Happy Meal, but you can steer them toward water as a beverage (instead of

Don't Be Tricked by Halloween Treats!

Halloween means candy and only a witch of a mom would ban the festivities entirely. You can navigate Halloween successfully. Just choose goodies carefully and limit your (and your little goblins') intake.

Best Picks

✓ Lollipops are great: They are satisfying and contain no fat and take a long time to eat. A Blowpop, for example, has 60 calories and 14 grams of carbohydrates.

✓ Remember Smarties? They have only 25 calories a roll. Two rolls of Smarties equal one Angel Carb on the Blueprint.

✓ Tootsie Rolls are a good low-fat option when you have a chocolate craving. But choose the small ones, which log in at 130 calories for 12. Another good choice is the mini York Peppermint Patty, which will cost you 50 calories or 100 for two.

✓ Rice Krispie Treats are now available in mini bars for Halloween: 2 bars are 90 calories and have 2 grams of fat.

Halloween Horrors

✓ Mounds pack a little mountain of calories—83—and a ton of saturated fat because of the coconut. A small, fun-size bar has 4 grams of saturated fat.

✓ A fun-size pack of M&M's has 105 calories, 5 grams of fat and 2.5 grams of saturated fat.

✓ Rollo's also came in high with 90 calories and 2.5 grams of fat for 3 little pieces!

✓ One fun-size Butterfinger has 100 calories and 4 grams of fat, with 2 grams of saturated fat.

soda) and an apple (instead of fries), or at least you can try to do so when they're small. Subway is always my favorite fast-food spot, because of its fresh fit for kids menu: They offer a healthy small sandwich, fruit and milk. See page 261 for details on which excellent choices I've found at a host of popular chains.

THE PANCAKE TRAP   If it's Saturday morning, it must be pancake time! It's great to have ritual breakfasts on a weekend when everyone is relaxed and family time is so special. But those whopping breakfasts can take a toll. A stack of pancakes with a giant side of bacon or sausage is not the light start to the weekend that you're looking for. I have a few suggestions for this situation. If you're a mom who's home with the kids all week, maybe it's dad's turn to spend some quality time with the little ones while you sleep late or even hit the gym or do an exercise video. If you'd feel robbed missing out on the gathering, then how about altering the recipes? You can find healthy pancake recipes with lots of fiber that, topped with fresh fruit or yogurt, make a delicious breakfast that everyone will enjoy. If you want to have something special for breakfast but you know that a pancake will set you off toward a Plunge, then consider something like Van's light waffles or a Vitatop muffin toasted with a Laughing Cow light cheese. These foods are a switch from your usual yogurt or hard-boiled eggs but they're still on the Blueprint and they're good, healthy choices that are a little more fun.

FAMILY EXERCISE   There's nothing like exercising with your kids to set a healthy example. When you have babies or toddlers your stroller can be your best friend. Whether you prefer a jogging stroller or a regular street stroller, a brisk walk with baby is one of the very best temptation killers possible. Research has actually shown (though I think it's just common sense!) that a ten-minute walk is probably the most effective technique for coping with food cravings.

If your kids are older, exercise with them. Go to the park, go for a walk, shoot some hoops, play Wii. I had a client who took her two sons swimming every winter Sunday at a hotel pool that was open to the public. They brought the Sunday newspaper and the adults read between swim time with the sons who loved that special routine.

SUMMER CAMP BLUBBER BLUES   If your child heads off to camp for the summer, it is not a license for you to go wild! Now, most of my clients find that when their children are away it's easier to stick to their diet and exercise routines because, for one thing, they simply have more hours in their day. But there are others, and you know who you are, who use the absence of the little ones to go on a total food binge. They either eat out too frequently or they plunge into carryout hell. It's very difficult to control your calorie intake when eating restaurant food. I have lots of tips on how to handle this in "Dine-Out Devils" (page 214), so take a good look at this section if you're tempted to throw all your weight loss progress to the winds while the kiddies munch s'mores.

THE EMPTY NEST   When the kids are gone, eating well can become easier in many respects. You don't need to stock the treats and carbs that the kids enjoy, and you usually can prepare lighter meals. But sometimes the loneliness of the empty nest can trigger Emotional Eating and sometimes the changed and perhaps reduced structure of your days can trigger Boredom Bingeing. Take a look at the strategies in both those Devil chapters.

Diet Devil #6
Boredom Bingeing

Boredom Bingeing is mindless eating in an endless, robotic loop. A handful of cereal and then, in an hour or so, some baby carrots. And then maybe a piece of cinnamon toast to get you to lunch, and a handful of chocolate chips because the bag was open. And so on and so on. All day long. Most Boredom Bingers are oblivious to their bites, picks and tastes. They feel that they eat pretty well. In fact, their meals might be models of healthy choices. But the constant nibbling that they often aren't even aware of adds a stream of calories in the course of the day that can add up to many extra pounds.

One of the questions I ask clients when I meet with them for the first time is, "Do you tend to lose weight on vacation?" If they answered yes, it usually means that they're Boredom Bingers. Boredom Bingers lose weight on vacation because when you're away there isn't a colleague's desk with an inviting bowl of M&M's. There's no pantry with half-empty sleeves of crackers. There are no plates to clear and pick off. There's no kitchen to close after dinner. In fact, there is no kitchen! For Boredom Bingers, eliminating these sources of mindless eating promotes reliable weight loss.

Are you hungry when you wake up? Are you hungry for

lunch or dinner? Most Boredom Bingers are rarely hungry. They've lost their sense of hunger and satiety because they're eating all the time. They're hardly conscious of what they're putting in their mouths, but they are orally fixated and they find it comforting to munch regularly throughout the day. Chewing is their background music. Many of my clients who are Boredom Bingers are ex-smokers. They like to have something in their mouths. They often tell me that they were thumb-suckers as children. Most people don't boredom binge at work because they're engrossed and busy. But stay-at-home moms, retirees, freelance workers—almost anyone who has regular long stretches of time at home—can struggle with Boredom Bingeing.

In my experience, three factors are involved in Boredom Binging: boredom (well duh!), stress and solitude. Here's another way to look at it:

> ➤ Time on your hands + something (anything)
> to feel anxious about + food in your
> kitchen = Boredom Bingeing!

We'll take a close look at remedies to the basic boredom issue below, but I want to highlight the second factor in Boredom Bingeing: Stress! As noted above, many people turn to mindless activities when stressed. Some people bite their nails. Some jiggle their foot. Some stuff cookies into their mouths at five-minute intervals until they can hardly breathe. If this last describes you, take a moment to examine what's causing the stress in your life. Is it a temporary situation like an illness or a problem with a child? Or is it something more permanent like a challenging job? Many people never connect the stress in their lives with the impulse to overeat. I had a client who had gained twenty pounds over the course of a year, and only when I questioned her did she finally connect her weight gain with her husband's job loss. Once she recognized what was prompting her to snack, she was better able to channel her anxiety and avoid overeating. If you suspect that stress plays a role in your Boredom Bingeing, take a look at Emotional Eating (p 113) for additional strategies.

Solitude—who knew it could be dangerous to your waistline? It's true, isn't it? You don't tend to eat a giant bag of M&M's when you're in a business meeting or at a PTA event. No, Boredom Bingers are closet eaters. It's those quiet moments alone when you let down your guard and head to the pantry. Unhealthy eating is often a guilty pleasure that you'd rather hide from others. Obviously you're always going to have time alone, but here's a good question to ask yourself: Would I eat this if my neighbor, my boss, my kid, my book group were watching? This question also forces you to look at whether you're really hungry.

Boredom Bingeing comforts you and distracts you from other things when you feel stressed. But here's something you know is true: Eating while bored does not make boredom go away and it's only a temporary comfort. Boredom Bingeing makes you less productive and even more stressed. In the long run, it's a habit that will make you feel out of control. And it's a habit you can definitely break using the strategies below. Ultimately, eating well strengthens your sense of control and it also promotes calm, clarity and the ability to be more productive.

I confess I can have my own struggles with Boredom Bingeing: Even as I was working on this section of the book I found myself picking mindlessly at a stale bag of seasoned nuts my husband must have collected a while back on a business trip. Eat, type, lick my fingers, eat, type. . . . How can I be doing exactly what I'm telling readers not to do?! And why does it feel so good to eat when we're bored or even trying to concentrate on something? Why is it that we never feel inclined to reach for a cucumber when stressed? It could have something to do with your levels of the stress hormone cortisol. People who secrete higher levels of cortisol in response to stress also tend to eat more food and food that is higher in carbs than those who have lower cortisol levels. So if you're more sensitive to stress, you might well be more likely to Boredom Binge.

Moreover, many of the foods that are our preferred snacking foods are loaded with sugar, fat and salt. This fat, sugar and salt stimulate our brains to release certain chemicals—dopamine and opioids—that motivate our behavior and make us want to eat more and more of the brain-satisfying foods, whether or not we are hungry. These foods thus become, in their way, addictive. So when you start to power through a bag of chips, it's hard to stop. In addition to the pleasure of the taste and the mouth feel and the delicious salty crunchiness of it, you're getting a bit of a buzz as you work your way down to those last crumbs. That's why this kind of eating is habit forming. It's so satisfying. But it's obvious what constant grazing at home does to your weight and your morale.

Now a rare Boredom Binge isn't a catastrophe. A snow day, a long weekend . . . we all occasionally have an unexpected situation that encourages us to believe that munching is the most interesting activity available. But if you find that you're *frequently* snacking for lack of something better to do, it's time to get control. It's the *habit* part of Boredom Bingeing that is the real problem. You will be able to determine if you are beleaguered by this Devil by checking out your food journal. If you recorded honestly and you're a Boredom Binger, you'll see a random list of food entries. Someone who has a problem with volume eating might have three giant meals a day, but the Boredom Binger may actually skip meals and instead list a host of bites, picks and tastes.

Are you a Boredom Binger? You'll know for sure once you complete the food diary I described in "Free-Style Dieting" (page 83).

Take a look at your honest record of what you ate in the course of a couple of days. Is your day sprinkled with snacks—the little tidbits, or bites, picks, tastes? Are you nibbling from sunrise to the evening news? If so, you are a Boredom Binger. (The Late-Night Shuffle, another Diet Devil, is all about eating after dinner [see page 99]; the Boredom Binger is typically a daytime eater.)

You do not have to be a hostage to Boredom Bingeing. Here are my top strategies that will help you conquer this Diet Devil.

What Boredom Bingers Need to Know

EMBRACE STRUCTURE If you're a Boredom Binger, it's critical to create structure in your day. If you are still in your pj's at 10:00 A.M., you're in trouble. More than any other Devil, Boredom Binging tempts those who are not in control of their time. Plan your day in advance. I think the best morning routine for those who are at home is exercise followed by shower followed by dressing followed by breakfast. A late-afternoon activity like yoga or walking the dog or errands gives you something to look forward to and helps you structure your time. Think ahead when it comes to meals. Always have healthy options on hand and a stash of healthy frozen dinners that you can dip into when necessary. Be sure to stock some frozen veggies like broccoli. I love the type where you can just toss the whole bag in the micro. See my shopping list for great suggestions on frozen meals and veggies.

LIVE THE BLUEPRINT If you tend to Boredom Binge, you need to make a decision that you will eat three healthy meals a day—no more; no less. Let the Blueprint be your guide. (The one exception is on weekends. If you get up late and skip breakfast then you're down to two meals that day. But there are guidelines in the Blueprint for that too.) If you have already figured out what you're going to be eating on a given day—maybe a Phase breakfast and a Phase lunch and, say, a healthy frozen dinner if you're staying in—you have already won the biggest battle of your diet day.

Regular meals at regular times is the backbone of the Blueprint and a critical component of healthy eating. It's especially important for Boredom Bingers. For one thing scheduled meals help you recognize hunger, and Boredom Bingers commonly need to reacquaint themselves with what it feels like to have that little pinch in their tummies that tells them it's time to eat. When you eat regularly, your body will come to expect a meal at a certain hour and you will begin to feel hungry for an hour or so before that meal. Don't skip meals. Because Boredom Bingers can be out of touch with hunger, they tend to skip meals, which only makes them more ravenous and less able to control themselves when they finally do eat. If you find yourself not particularly hungry at mealtime, just eat lightly.

KEEP A CLEAN KITCHEN   If you're like most of my clients you can probably instantly identify any tempting goodies that are hiding at the back of your cupboard. That half box of cookies? Right behind the flour. The remaining chocolate chips from that recipe you made last spring? At the bottom of the spice drawer. Am I right? You know the answer to this but you keep avoiding it—empty your kitchen of all tempting junky nibbling food, the kind that calls to you in the night. Be honest with yourself and get a great big garbage bag and toss all your temptations. I know it's hard, but if your goal is to lose weight and feel great in your clothes, it's worth it. (One client told me that after she tossed all her junk food, she felt like she'd already lost five pounds!) Don't trick yourself into buying treats while you're feeling strong. We all have our power moments when we feel we could easily turn our backs on temptation.

But remember that when you're feeling low or bored, you're a whole different animal. And, by the way, never shop for groceries when you're hungry or feeling blue. But you already knew that, right? If you must keep something on hand for a loved one, ask them to hide it for you. This works for my husband's secret stash of peanut butter. Or, if you do need to buy treats for your kids, pick something that doesn't appeal to you.

MANAGE SNACKS   Boredom Bingers have to take their snacks seriously. No whimsical "Should I have some crackers this afternoon?" for you! Do you need a snack? Here's how to find out: If you find that eating a single afternoon snack helps you eat less at dinner or helps keep you from Boredom Bingeing in the afternoon, then you need a snack. If a snack has no real effect on the amount of food you eat in a given day, then it is probably unnecessary. If you need a snack, it's important to build one into your day because it will really help you to stay on track. The best afternoon snacks are hand fruits—that is, fruit that fits in your hand—like an apple, orange or small banana. Even a small grapefruit can be a good option. If fruit doesn't do the trick for you, try two FiberRich or GG crackers with one Laughing Cow light cheese.

DELAY MEALS   We've all been told that we should eat when we wake up. For some of us, especially those who are controlled in their eating habits, this is true. But for those who are Boredom Bingers, an early breakfast can trigger excess consumption. Especially if you're not even hungry for that breakfast. I tell my Boredom Bingers to try to delay their breakfast until the latest time that they can comfortably eat. Don't go past 10:30, but if you're comfortable having your breakfast at 10:00 A.M., that's fine. The later you push back breakfast, the later you can have lunch and then dinner. The exception to this advice is for people in high-stress jobs who start very early in the morning. These people can get so caught up in their work that they forget breakfast entirely. If this is you, don't delay breakfast; eat early. Put a sticker on your desk to remind you to order lunch by 11:00 so you'll be sure to have it delivered before you're ravenous. Your afternoon snack, if you need one, is later too. On weekends, many of my clients sleep late and enjoy just two meals. This delaying strategy takes advantage of avoiding food at times that you're not hungry and helping you relearn what it feels like to be hungry in the first place.

CONDENSE YOUR EATING TIME   There's a difference between eating slowly and lingering over your food. Slow eating (as opposed to Hoovering) is good; lingering is bad. Boredom Bingers tend to linger. I learned early on that certain clients could make a cracker snack last an hour and a half as they bit off teeny tiny nibbles. Same with meals: They could turn a grilled chicken breast and stalk of broccoli into an eating marathon. I think we do this because we simply want to make the pleasure last. But when you're trying to lose weight, it's a mistake. You really don't want to be eating all day because this interferes with your ability to develop a healthy hunger in preparation for your next meal. Most meals should take no longer than sixty minutes max (unless it's a special night out or a gala event) and most snacks should be eaten in about twenty minutes.

FOCUS ON YOUR FOOD   You're rushing to get out the door in the morning. You're trying to get dressed, you're carrying around a yogurt, talking to your sister on the phone, firing off e-mails, opening an old bill you just found in the rubble. . . . Are you tasting that breakfast? Is it satisfying you? Do you even remember eating it? Frankly, I think that trying to tell people not to multitask while eating is sort of hopeless these days. It's like telling people they can never drink wine or put any milk in their coffee. Who lives that way? But, and it's a big "but," when you ignore what you're eating, you tend to eat too much. Eating on autopilot is a waste of calories. If you're shoving in your breakfast while dressing, it's perhaps time to consider waiting and enjoying your breakfast a bit later in the morning, at a time when you can really focus on what you're eating and enjoy it. For some people that might mean eating at the office or after the kids have been dropped off at school. And I do suggest putting away your smartphone for mealtime. There's no work e-mail that can't wait until you've finished a meal. I think that people are inclined to consume more calories when they're listening to their e-mail box pinging every few seconds. That sound increases anxiety and can trigger an appetite surge. Conscious eating is what I'm encouraging. If you make an effort to focus on your food, you'll enjoy what you're eating and you'll feel like you've had a meal! Moreover, you'll recognize when you're full and you'll probably eat less.

BECOME A PHASE EATER   Anything that makes you think—or obsess—about food throughout the day is counterproductive. This is why some diets ultimately fail—you think about nothing but your next meal, day in and day out, until you *must eat*, now! Thinking about food makes you hungry, right? This is also why those diets that have you eating eight times a day can be counterproductive. Remember Phase Eating in the FreeStyle Diet Devil section? It's about picking one breakfast and one lunch and having it for a week or two or even three. There's nothing wrong with eating a small carton of yogurt with some cereal mixed in and a piece of fruit for breakfast every morning for weeks on end if you enjoy it. Same goes for lunch—a turkey sandwich on whole wheat bread with a slather of mustard and some nice crunchy lettuce is a great lunch. You may want to vary your dinners, but it's good to keep a selection of healthy frozen dinners on hand for those times when you can't bear the thought of cooking. Of course if you get tired of your Phase choices, it's time to move on to something else. Check my Sample Menus (page 50) for lots of good meal suggestions.

WATER, WATER, WATER   Boredom Bingers are often lazy water drinkers, and when we get lazy about water consumption, the munchies and mindless eating may dominate. Many people disregard the advice to drink plenty of water because they've heard it so many times and it seems so simple . . . how could it make a difference? Well, let me tell you that I've had so many clients in the past ten years who were model eaters and just couldn't budge the needle on the scale until I insisted they up their water intake. Bingo: The weight invariably came off. Nobody knows for certain why serious water consumption works to speed weight loss, but here are my theories:

➤ It's quite possible that there's a metabolic shift when water intake is increased and thus promotes weight loss.

➤ When you drink water, your stomach has something in it and you're less hungry. (We've all heard the advice to drink water before a meal or a party and it works!)

➤ We often dine outside the home these days, and too many of these meals are salt fests. Your body can better tolerate salt when it's well hydrated.

➤ More water means less bloat. When you're less bloated, you feel better and the better you feel, the easier it is to stay on track.

➤ If you follow my guidelines and drink 8 cups of water a day, it's difficult to squeeze in the coffees and other drinks that add up in calories.

My guideline is LBL, a liter by lunch. Focus on drinking that first liter—4 cups—before lunch. You should get the second liter in before dinner. Any water beyond that is a bonus.

SET YOUR START TIME   Feel the urge to wander into the kitchen for a handful of something? What time is it? Late afternoon is prime snack time for my clients. If you feel that restless urge to consume something, anything, at 3:00 or 4:00 P.M., make a decision: If you really need a snack, set a time to enjoy it. For many people 4:00 P.M. is good, or, if you're not eating dinner until after 7:00, then 4:30 or 5:00 P.M. might work for your snack. Settle on that time and then put the snack out of your mind until then. You don't really have to set a timer, but you can if you find it helps. Some snackers put a sticky note on their computer or fridge to remind them of their snack time. Setting up these guidelines for yourself frees you from agonizing about food and allows you to concentrate on the things you'd rather be doing. Also, you'll notice that if you plan an afternoon snack it can really help you avoid that mindless binge that can occur just before dinner and that spoils your appetite and packs in too many extra calories.

AVOID THE POPPABLE, PICKABLE, DIPPABLE, UNSTOPPABLE It's not always about calories! Sometimes it's about food that's just too easy to eat. Poppable foods are at the top of my must-avoid list. You can guess what they are: a giant barrel of pretzel nuggets, boxes of cereal big enough to live in and the bag of Halloween candy you confiscated from your child. And don't forget popcorn, chips and the stale seasoned nuts I mentioned earlier. But even foods that seem to be healthy can be too poppable to risk. Like cherry tomatoes, olives, dried fruit, wasabi peas, nuts, baby carrots, grapes and even raw veggies dipped into hummus. A cup of hummus and a cucumber can add up to a 500-calorie snack that would take about five miles of running to burn off. It's really best to free your kitchen of poppables. Make a clean sweep of it.

BAN THE MISHMOSH DINNER   The Mishmosh dinner is not a meal; it's a random, unplanned munch-fest. It is often the culmination of a Boredom Bingeing day—one where there were no regular meals but a mindless parade of snacks. So now it's near dinnertime and you're not at all hungry. So you figure you'll just have a couple of rice cakes with peanut butter. And then, an hour later, there's the FiberRich cracker with a Laughing Cow light cheese because that's a healthy choice. And then some steamed broccoli and a few more rice cakes. And maybe just one chicken nugget. This whole festival takes up a couple of hours of your evening as you cycle in and out of the kitchen, trying to come to grips with dinner. The solution to the Mishmosh dinner is a frozen dinner. Even a frozen dinner with more calories than you'd like is far, far better than the open-ended calorie load of a Mishmosh dinner.

KEEP BUSY   You never Boredom Binge when you're busy. Haven't you had days or at least afternoons when you've been so busy that you haven't given a thought to food? When you're surprised that it's already an hour past lunchtime? That's one of the key strategies to break the Boredom Bingeing habit: Keep busy! I know, I know . . . this sounds so obvious. But really, think about it: If you have lots of unstructured time you are going to be tempted to eat. And if you feel bored, it's a sign that you need to make changes in your life. Most of the time, boredom is a signal that you need some kind of change. Maybe not major changes; maybe just creating a to-do list that will keep you occupied in your downtime. Does your garden need a spot check? Are your closets ready for their close-up? If you are sitting in a chair on Saturday afternoon being bored, you're going to eat. If you are cleaning out the garage, you're going to burn calories! So get busy. You'll feel more positive and you'll avoid Boredom Bingeing.

A NOTE TO GUM CHEWERS AND CANDY SUCKERS Do you chew more than one pack of gum or more than ten pieces of sucking candy a day? Many Boredom Bingers used to be smokers and adopted the habit of chewing candy and sucking gum in an effort to stop smoking. Other Boredom Bingers just enjoy having something in their mouths at all times. How could this affect weight loss? Well, a pack of gum can add up to 150 calories and popping sugar candies could add up to way more (to say nothing of the cavities!). Sometimes simply cutting out this habit can lead to weight loss because of the reduced calories. Plus sugar can lead to more cravings and could ultimately lead to poor food choices throughout the day. Even sugar-free gum and candies can pose a problem: For one thing, constant chewing is a habit you want to break. For another there are recent studies linking excess artificial sweeteners to a slowed metabolism and insulin spikes that can cause difficulty in losing weight as well as energy slumps throughout the day. Artificial sweeteners can also cause gas and bloating. While occasional pieces of sugar-free gum and candies are fine, the regular daily habit of constant chewing is where trouble begins.

FIND ACTIVITY TREATS Not all treats have to be edible! And sometimes you don't want to keep busy by cleaning a closet or vacuuming the living room. So figure out a few activities that you enjoy, that give you real pleasure. If you're working at home, you really do need to take a break now and again—one that doesn't involve a trip to the kitchen. If a walk outside doesn't appeal, then spend a half hour with your favorite magazine or a novel. Or call a friend. Surely there's someone who would love to hear from you. One of my clients told me she buys pretty cards at museums and every now and again when she's thinking of hitting the kitchen she pulls one out and writes a "thinking of you" note to a friend. Everything is so electronic these days that a handwritten and posted note is a real treat. And by the time she's finished with the note the urge to snack has passed.

AVOID WORKPLACE MUNCHIES   It's not only stay-at-homes who Boredom Binge. Have you ever wandered through your office, searching for the proverbial bowls of candy and other goodies that the office devils have put out for you? You can pretend that you're just getting a drink at the water cooler, but you know in your heart you're scavenging for tidbits. If this describes you, the solutions include some of those previously mentioned, including popping a breath strip or sugarless gum or candy before wandering or else simply relying on your water bottle for frequent oral gratification. Stick a slice of lemon or lime in your water and that citrus flavor will help ward off the longing for sweets.

AVOID TRIGGER FOODS   Most of us have foods that just set us off on a munching binge. Whether it's a chip or a bowl of cherries, recognize the foods that are your trigger foods and get rid of them. Keep them out of your kitchen and your life. You really have to make this decision at the supermarket: Don't buy foods that you know are going to be difficult to resist. It's easier to eliminate these foods from your kitchen than to be constantly struggling with temptation.

THINNER ON MONDAY   I've had so many clients tell me that they can do well during the week but the weekend just becomes a calorie binge. There are pancake breakfasts with the family, fatty brunches with friends, endless snacking, dinners out and a Sunday night football game with wings and guac, until they morph into a total pig in a blanket. It's Boredom Bingeing at its worst. Don't let it happen to you! With a little planning you can face Monday morning with a smile and your skinny pants. Monday is a tough day for most of us anyhow: The weekend is over and adding a couple of pounds in a couple of days just makes everything more depressing. So your new goal is thinner on Monday! If you can stick to my strategies and wake up lighter on Monday morning, you can break the cycle that most of us get stuck on: Lose all week; reverse and gain on the weekend.

As we all know, nothing says relax like Friday night. But it's important to start the weekend strong. Don't let things fall apart when the lure of two days of relaxation dissolves your willpower. If you wake up feeling fat and awful on Saturday morning, it's going to be a struggle to eat well over the weekend. A fat Saturday is going to prompt you to abandon hope and dive into a pile of pancakes. Be sure you have the makings of a healthy breakfast on hand so that even if you do make a pancake meal for the kids you can enjoy your own lean, healthy choices. It's especially important to plan ahead on the weekend: Look ahead to any meals that are already scheduled—dinner with friends, a social brunch—and think about how to spend your calories.

While it's important to stick to the Blueprint for the first three weeks, after that time you can be a little more flexible; many of my clients will choose to have one carb weekdays but will allow themselves two on the weekend days. The critical goal is to maintain control. You need to know yourself: If one indulgence is going to set you off toward a binge, then skip it. But if you know that you can control yourself, allow that indulgence with these three guidelines: It has to be with other people, it has to be a normal serving (no boxes of cupcakes or warehouse-size bag of chips) and it should be in the evening, at dinner.

EMPLOY A DENTAL DIVERSION   Here are two tips that clients have passed along to me: One woman told me that she always keeps those little dental floss thingies near her sofa and her desk. When she's home alone she just flosses away while watching TV or surfing the Internet. She claims it's saved her thousands of calories. Another tactic is to simply brush your teeth. When you have that clean feeling in your mouth, you're less likely to want to eat. I've always found this effective.

EXERCISE   Now I'm not talking about rushing to the gym for a class or jogging for a mile or two. Though there's nothing wrong with those options either. I'm simply suggesting the equivalent of a quick jolt of electricity—like a restart—to change your inclination from Boredom Bingeing to healthy, productive activity. It might amount to five sit-ups or a few vigorous stretches. My clients tell me that they're amazed at how effective this little exercise boost can be. It gets the blood pumping and, for most people, short-circuits their lust for crumb cake. Check out "Sloth," page 161, for some good exercise tips.

SUCCUMB   When all else fails and you really, truly, absolutely must eat something, here are the acceptable choices:

> ➤ Cut-up cucumbers

> ➤ Sliced peppers

> ➤ Celery

> ➤ Sliced turkey

> ➤ Cooked egg whites

Diet Devil #7
Sloth

I have two types of clients. Some exercise already, maybe not consistently, but they have made exercise a part of their lives. Some, in fact, are devoted exercisers. If this describes you, great! You don't really need to worry too much about this Diet Devil. Keep up your exercise, and read this section primarily to learn what I've found to be the most effective exercises. If, however, you've spent years trudging on a treadmill at the same easy speed—and never lost an ounce—you may be a "lazy exerciser." If you want to see real results on the scale, it's time to revise your exercise program.

Many of my clients, on the other hand, are committed nonexercisers. Some are just so overscheduled and busy and stressed that the mention of the word "exercise" makes them want to run out and devour a bag of doughnut munchkins. Others have tried and failed. Maybe they gave up after a couple of painful spin classes. Maybe their favorite yoga instructor moved on. Maybe they found that exercise made them so hungry that they actually *gained* weight. (Talk about a frustrating setback!)

If you're a nonexerciser, Sloth is having its evil way with you. I'm going to show you how you can beat this Devil and supercharge your weight loss. But not at some triathlete marathon speed—at *your* speed!

Now, before you get anxious and protest, "I just can't/won't exercise," know that I'm not suggesting that you jump on a treadmill this afternoon. No, my years of experience working with thousands of clients prove that while exercise is important, *diet is more so.* If I had to break it down to a percentage, I'd say that losing weight is 90% what you eat and 10% exercise. Alternative theories are in the minority, but it is irrefutable that *you're not going to lose weight if you don't work on what you eat.* Healthy food choices mean weight loss. This has always been a controversial topic, but recent research backs me up. Look at it this way: If you weigh about 150 pounds it takes about an hour of high impact aerobics to burn off as little as 500 calories. That's approximately two slices of cheese pizza. So my most important message about exercise is this: Even if you just hate the thought of exercising, you can still lose weight. Food comes first; moving comes second.

Now I've waited to mention this not because it's not important but because perhaps you've heard it before. But it does bear repeating. Exercise can really help you when it comes to healthy weight loss. For one thing, exercise is a key player in leading a healthier, longer and happier life. It relieves stress, helps with weight control, lowers your risk for chronic diseases such as heart disease, colon cancer and type 2 diabetes, helps control blood pressure and improves self-esteem by reducing feelings of depression and anxiety. And if these benefits haven't convinced you, consider that it will also increase your fitness level, build and maintain bones, muscles and joints, develop endurance and strength and enhance flexibility and posture.

Now, let me confess that I'm a serious exerciser. I grew up in a family of runners and I just don't feel good if I don't exercise. I believe that exercise is important for a host of reasons. For me, it's not only critical for stress relief, but it also simply makes me feel good about myself and more in control of my life. In fact, I get up early—really early some days—and run

Isabel's Story

Isabel came to me as a totally committed nonexerciser who had twenty-five pounds to lose. "I was so relieved when I had my first meeting with Heather and she didn't talk about exercise. I'm a teacher with three of my own kids at home, so my days are full. And teaching is physically exhausting sometimes. Believe me, the last thing I ever wanted to do was exercise, and I was so nervous on that first visit that Heather would pressure me to get busy with the spandex. Well a month goes by and I really began to see results. Following Heather's eating recommendations, I'd lost eight pounds in those first weeks and my clothes were all getting loose. I was really beginning to believe that maybe I could get to my goal. Up till then, Heather still hadn't said anything about exercise, and I was beginning to think it was odd because of course you always hear so much about how important it is in weight loss. So I finally told Heather that I thought maybe it might be a good idea if I started to work out a little. Well, she smiled at me like she'd been waiting for me to ask that question for three weeks! I joined a gym and began going three times a week. I had my sitter stay a little later and sometimes I went in the evening after my husband was home to watch the kids. I was really surprised at how exercising made it easier to eat well. It reinforced the good feelings I got from losing weight in the first place. I know I'm going to get to my goal and no one is more surprised than me that I'm now a regular exerciser."

along the Hudson River path and across Central Park to my office. (I wash up and change at the office.) I don't do this every day but as often as I can. It helps me get my day off to a great start and it makes whatever I have to face seem more manageable. You don't have to be a runner, and you don't have to be a gym rat. But it's helpful to learn which types of exercise are best for weight loss. I'll give you pointers on that, and I'll give

> **Big Fat Fact**
>
> Years of experience have taught me that clients who only diet and skip exercise will only get so far in weight loss. Those who diet first and then start exercising have faster and more long-lasting results than nonexercisers.

you some suggestions on how you might squeeze activity into your life.

I never tell nonexercisers that they have to start exercising. And yet almost every single one of them comes to me after two or three weeks on my Blueprint and asks about when and how they should start doing some exercising. Why? Because they start to lose weight and they begin to feel, maybe for the first time in a long time, good about themselves. They're in control. They're ready to take more on. It's always a happy day for me when someone walks out of my office resolved to start exercising because I know it means that they're ready to blast on through to their goal. I also know that exercise is going to make it easier for them to stick to their guns when it comes to healthy eating.

What Victims of Sloth Need to Know

FIRST, ADJUST TO THE BLUEPRINT   If you don't already exercise, wait a week or two on the Blueprint before you begin. Why? Exercise takes energy in the form of calories. In other words, it makes you hungry. You don't want to begin a new, healthy-eating plan and find that you're starving. Give your body a chance to lose a few pounds and adjust to a lower food intake before you put another stress on it. There's another reason to delay exercising: You don't want to overload yourself with new demands and risk discouragement. I've had clients rush into major life reforms that include a diet, an exercise program and everything from a closet-cleaning binge to a total body exfoliation only to find after a few days that they just can't sustain their good intentions. So don't overload yourself: First the Blueprint; then get moving!

JUST GET OFF YOUR BUTT!   Some people keep putting off any exercise because they make it too complicated. Don't know what to choose, don't know what to wear, don't know how long to do it. . . . Conquer this crazy Devil of indecision! Pick an activity that will fit into your lifestyle. It can be as simple as fast walking in your neighborhood. Many of my clients start out just like that: a brisk walk early in the morning or evening. Anyone can manage that. Try to fit in a workout daily—or at least three times a week—and then both weekend days (almost everyone has more time on weekends). If you prefer a gym, try fast walking on a treadmill or using the elliptical, a bike or stair climber. The point is to get your heart rate up. If you're chatting on your cell phone the whole time, you're not working hard enough.

Exercise and the Food Journal

Don't forget to record your exercise in your food journal. It helps keep you honest. In the beginning you can just record the activity and duration. As time goes on you may want to record intensity, using information from your heart monitor or whatever helps you keep on track. Most people find that when they jot down their exercise, they're more likely to work it into their day.

CARDIO FIRST   In general, I think it's best for beginner exercisers to start with cardiovascular exercise. That means running, walking, Stairmaster, elliptical . . . anything that gets your heart rate up. Some people jump in with weights first and while there is some argument for weights—it's easy to do at home, for example—I think that, in the beginning, cardio is more effective for weight loss. While it's true that the muscles you build with weight training do burn more calories throughout the day, without cardio you're just building muscles with fat on top. My recommendation is to start shedding the fat first with cardio and then build in weight training. If you have a lot of weight to lose, then it's best to stick to nonimpact cardio—the elliptical, stationery bike, or swimming—to prevent injury.

CHOOSE AN EXERCISE THAT HELPS CONTROL YOUR APPETITE
When you do begin to exercise, say, after your second week on the Blueprint, choose an activity that won't boost your appetite in a major way. There's no hard-and-fast rule on what to choose; everybody's metabolism is a little different. I've had clients who were able to eat well while doing spinning classes, but as soon as they started to run they became ravenous. I've had others who tell me that when they do cardio, they can't stick to the Blueprint. Nevertheless, I usually recommend some type of cardio to begin, since it seems to work best for most people. When you get to within five or ten pounds of your goal weight, you can add weight training or something like Pilates. If you find that your exercise is causing you to feel noticeably hungrier, then switch it up. You might want to try yoga or perhaps weight training instead of the elliptical. Tune in to what your body is telling you. There's no perfect exercise formula and everybody really is different. You want exercise to make you feel more conscious of your body, more in control and better able to eat well. If it's making you hungry, find an alterna-

tive activity. Exercise needs to be your ally and, with the right choice, it can be your best diet friend.

THE TWENTY-MINUTE RULE   Most of my clients bite off more than they can chew, and that holds for exercise too. They are enthusiastic and ambitious only to become discouraged when they can't stick to their goal. My advice is to start with a twenty-minute goal. All you have to do is move your legs for twenty minutes. And I've found that almost everyone, if they shoot for twenty minutes, will do at least a half hour! Your ultimate goal is thirty to forty-five minutes of moderate to vigorous daily physical activity for a recommended five times a week. I know this may seem excessive, especially if your goal is just to start going to the gym again, but you can build up to it. All that matters is that you get started. Don't overwhelm yourself. Remember, no one's judging you.

LAZY EXERCISING!   Remember those people I mentioned who cover miles weekly on the treadmill but never lose one ounce? It's important to remember that exercising is about intensity. Too many of us head to the gym, put on our headphones for music and set the treadmill for that same old comfortable pace for the same old comfortable time. Research shows that it is not just the *duration* of your exercise that counts but also the *intensity*, especially when you're trying to lose weight. You want to try to target your heart rate at 65% for as long as you can and to maximize your heart rate with an aerobic push at 85% at least once. (It is impossible to maintain this heart rate for a long time; it usually lasts for about thirty seconds. Use the formulas below to calculate yours.) Hitting these target heart rates is considered vigorous physical activity. To keep track of your heart rate, invest in a heart rate monitor once you've really committed to an exercise routine. Before I discovered a heart rate monitor, my running was completely haphazard. It was amazing how motivating it was to strap on that monitor and assess how I'd performed on each run. There's lots of information available online and elsewhere on good brands to choose.

➤ 65% intensity = (220 − [age]) × 0.65
➤ 85% intensity = (220 − [age]) × 0.85

BANISH THE MAÑANA DEVIL   Try your best to exercise in the morning. You know why—if you don't get it done first thing, it often doesn't happen. You can always *make* more time in the morning by simply getting up earlier. You only need twenty minutes to a half hour of exercise to start, and most people can manage to fit that in before his or her day begins. There's an additional benefit to morning exercise: When you exercise on an empty stomach, you tend to burn fat rather than the fast-energy sugars that you'd burn after eating. As for me, I plan my day so that exercise is automatic. I really think that, for most people, it's the only way to make it work.

DON'T TRADE GYM TIME FOR PIG OUTS   I don't believe in exercising to eat. I've had so many clients tell me that they do 45 minutes or 90 minutes or 120 minutes of cardio daily, and they figure that helps them burn X number of calories and therefore they can eat a slice of pizza a day with no consequences. These people love to see the "calories burned" figure on the treadmill because they're translating that number into a big fat greasy "reward." Well, nutrition is a science but it's not exact. Research says that it takes cutting out 3,500 calories for someone to lose a pound. But I've seen people who make one simple change in their diet, like eliminating an 80-calorie afternoon snack, and lose two pounds in a week. This won't happen for everyone but I have actually seen it with some clients. So while it's true that weight loss is about calories taken in versus calories spent, it's not a simple equation. We all know people who claim they eat a light, healthy diet, spend an hour a day on the treadmill and never lose an ounce. Sometimes excess salt in the treats is a problem. Sometimes it's the high fat content. Sometimes it's just the mystery of your individual metabolism. So don't get into the mind-set that you'll be able to afford unhealthy treats if you exercise. And, by the way, if you were an avid exerciser and stopped for some reason, you may be shocked at how quickly you can gain weight. It's important to adjust your calorie intake to compensate for your reduced activity.

A NOTE TO EX-ATHLETES   Were you ever an athlete? I've had clients who were once athletes—marathon runners, college athletes, serious skiers, tennis players—who had stopped exercising for one reason or another (usually because of time constraints). This is a mistake because these people really need to exercise for both mental and physical fitness. If you were once an athlete who's now struggling with weight, it's important to figure out a way to get back in the game. No need to wait a few weeks to begin. Just start slowly to avoid injury. Whether it's the gym, regular games like tennis or squash or, like me, simply getting up early and running, just do it! It will give a significant boost to your weight loss campaign and your morale.

A MARATHON WILL NOT MAKE YOU THIN   This is a Devil that I encounter every year in New York. Clients come to me all in a frenzy and say, "I'm training for the marathon and I've never weighed more!" Counterintuitive, right? Well, the truth is that when you're running for miles, you're experiencing a major appetite boost. You're burning a ton of calories, after all! Moreover, when you exercise really heavily you tend to overindulge in the wrong types of food: doughnuts anyone? So if you're training for a strenuous event, great. But don't expect to lose a great deal of weight just because of all that exercise. And try to focus on eating healthy foods rather than telling yourself you can "afford" to eat all those extra goodies. I'm all for eating carbs like turkey sandwiches, sushi rolls, sweet potatoes, brown rice and other Angel Carbs, but the "carb loading" that involves mountains of pasta is not the answer.

DANCE, DANCE, DANCE!   There are people who just hate the idea of exercise. They abhor the gym. They don't want to lift anything heavier than their grocery bags. If this describes you, dancing may be your activity of choice. Enthusiastic dancing can burn as many calories as jogging or cycling, and it can be done at a gym or community center or even in your living room. *Dance, Dance Revolution* is a popular music video game that will keep you on your toes.

A NOTE ON INJURIES AND SURGERIES   I've worked with many clients who have had an injury or surgery, and while they're recovering, they just pile on the food. If you were active and became inactive due to injury or surgery, you're vulnerable to weight gain. But this is the perfect time to focus solely on your diet. Think of your clean diet as your new exercise. If you've been relying primarily on exercise for weight control, you'll soon see how powerful and how important a healthy diet can be.

Exercise Basics

BEGINNER: Start with three days a week and get in thirty minutes of vigorous exercise (walking on the treadmill or using the elliptical, bike or stair climber).

ALREADY EXERCISING: Boost your exercise from three to five days a week. Consider investing in a heart rate monitor.

ALREADY EXERCISING FIVE DAYS: You may already be doing just fine. Make sure to adjust your activity to your caloric intake so you can enjoy continued weight loss. If your activity level makes you hungry, consider reducing your energy expenditure to see if it has any affect on your appetite.

Top Starter Tips for Beginning Exercisers

➤ If you're joining a gym, choose one that makes you feel comfortable. I have had clients who joined gyms and then were discouraged because everyone there was a skinny-minny spandex queen. If going to the gym is going to make you feel bad about yourself, it's not going to help. Find one that's welcoming and has an atmosphere that makes you feel at home. Even if you have to travel just a bit more, it will be worth it.

➤ No time for the gym? Consider killing two birds with one stone by working exercise into your commute. As I've mentioned, I've gotten in the habit of running to or from work. Biking or waking up a bit early for a brisk walk to work can also do the trick. If you can't walk all the way, you can plan to get off the bus or subway a few stops early and make the rest of the trip at a brisk walk. Regardless, aim for about thirty minutes of a moderate to vigorous cardio workout. Just fifteen minutes in the morning and fifteen minutes in the evening gets you to your goal!

➤ Consider a personal trainer. Sometimes it's just too hard to get started all on your own. It's also extremely helpful to have an expert guide you through the best exercise routines to suit your physical condition and your schedule. If this might be a strain on your budget, bear in mind that you don't have to rely on a trainer for a long time: Sometimes just a few sessions to get you started are all you need. (A few sessions with a trainer make a terrific gift for a friend or loved one who's eager to start exercising!)

➤ Keep yourself entertained during the workout. This can be anything from creating an energizing playlist on your iPod or mp3 player, watching your favorite TV show, using Wii *Fit* or downloading a personal training track to your iPod. If you are one of those people who hate repetition or gets bored on the treadmill, take a dance class. Keeping yourself engaged will make the workout more fun and will make you more likely to stick with it.

➤ When you miss the gym one day—which is inevitable— don't fret. There are a multitude of activities you can do right in the comfort of your own home. Consider dips or ab work while watching TV, walking lunges around your living room or running up and down flights of stairs. If you are ever faced with the choice of an elevator or stairs, always opt for the stairs!

➤ Intervals are key! Interval training—exercise that involves bursts of high-energy activity alternating with slower movement—is a proven method for reaching your maximum heart rate. Most cardio machines now have an interval option, but there are also gym classes that incorporate this type of training. You can also do intervals yourself: Sprint for thirty seconds, walk or jog for one minute and repeat for up to thirty minutes.

➤ Mix it up! When motivation flags or your muscles get into a rut, you can change the intensity of your exercise or change the type of exercise. If you're a runner, try the elliptical or the Stairmaster. Take a spin class, a weight training class, a dance class, yoga or Pilates. These teachers are trained to keep you engaged and to motivate you. Yoga is also a great way to tighten your abs and strengthen your back muscles, which are hard to strengthen and often get overlooked.

➤ It's nice to know that these days you don't always have to join a gym: You can pick and choose among independent exercise classes. This is great if you don't want to commit to a monthly membership at a gym.

➤ Don't forget about weight training. If you have a gym membership, don't forget to check out the classes. Many gyms have classes that include weight circuit sessions or weights and many gym memberships include complementary training sessions that you may have passed up. You should aim to do weights two to three times a week to build and strengthen your muscles. I target my biceps, triceps and shoulders since those are used least in cardio workouts. And don't be afraid to use the machines, which can be fun.

➤ Change the channel . . . to the exercise channel on your TV. There are great exercising tips and new exercises that will keep your workout fresh.

➤ Lay out your clothes! If you're going to exercise in the morning, get everything ready the night before. I learned my lesson after missing too many morning runs because I couldn't find my socks or sports bra. Now I lay out both my workout and work clothes the night before. If you're planning to exercise after work: Pack your bag. If you get up intending to exercise in the morning but you can't find your leggings or your top or appropriate workout shoes, it's just too easy to give up. Moreover, seeing those clothes all ready for you is a great reminder to get moving. If you've already made the effort to set out your clothes, you might as well hop to it!

➤ Gotta Love Lululemon. Whether it's Lululemon leggings for women or Under Armour for men, invest in workout clothes that make you feel good. And this includes your workout socks, shoes, undies and sports bras. It may seem silly, but wearing great clothes to exercise in will improve your workout. Baggy clothes weigh you down, get in the way and make you feel like a schlump.

➤ Sip don't gulp. Make sure you hydrate thirty minutes prior to your workout but only sip your water during it. Also, don't eat within thirty minutes of beginning exercise. I tell clients not to count the water they drink during or right after exercise as part of their two daily liters. That's because it's sweated right out.

➤ Stretch!! I know you want to race out of the gym, but you need to cool down your muscles. Be sure to take five minutes at the end of your workout to stretch. This will also improve your flexibility!

Diet Devil #8
Celebrations! Vacations!

Why is it always easy to lose weight at a spa? Or the hospital? Or in prison? When your food arrives on a tray in little portion-controlled blocks and your days are spent getting massages or breaking rocks and there are no nearby candy dishes or chocolate bunnies or cupcakes . . . well, who couldn't stick to any old eating plan? But of course you don't live that way and, really (except for the spa), who would want to? No, you have the pleasures and challenges of birthday parties, Christmas, vacation trips, weddings, and girls' night out to deal with. And thank goodness! Girls, and everyone else, definitely want to have fun. But fun too often translates into food, and lots of it. So I'm going to share with you my best techniques for avoiding calorie blowouts while still partying down.

Many of us manage to stick to our healthy resolutions in the routine circumstances of our everyday lives, but when something out of the ordinary is on the calendar, especially if it revolves around food, the Celebration Devils can come out in full force. Celebration and Vacation Devils convince us that we can cut loose from healthy eating because . . . well, because these events are exceptions. Plus, we deserve it! Well, not quite. We really don't deserve to be dissatisfied with our weight, so let's take a close look at Celebrations and Vacations and see how we can enjoy them without guilt.

Here's the bare-bones truth: Many people use any excuse to go hog wild, whether a casual lunch with an old friend or a grand twenty-fifth anniversary trip to Paris. We tell ourselves it's "just this once," but it's not. Almost every week of the year has some occasion to tempt us to shrug off our resolutions. While it's definitely important to have occasions in your life where weight loss isn't at the top of your to-do list, they should be unusual.

Maybe my client Jed's comments on the Celebration Devil will sound familiar:

When I came to see Heather I was totally discouraged about my weight. I was really good at losing a few pounds but it seemed that every single time I made a little progress some event would come along and trip me up. The last time this happened I had a single week where there was an engagement party for my sister and then I had to entertain out-of-town clients and that Sunday was the Super Bowl. I ended that week right back at my original weight and wiped out all the gains I'd made in the previous three weeks. My problem was that I compartmentalized my eating: I was either "on a diet" or I was doing something special and that meant I wasn't "on a diet." Heather helped me see my eating in a more holistic way. It's not about being "on a diet." She helped me recognize that my life is likely to be rich in events, parties and celebrations but that very few, if any, of them are once-in-a-lifetime occasions requiring overindulgence. Now I've become more strategic about my choices and I eat pretty well all the time. When I'm doing something special I might allow myself more leeway but it's never a total blowout. In fact, I'm closing in on my target weight. I don't think I'll ever be back in my "circus pants" now that I know how to roll with the party punches.

Jed's story is instructive, and I hope it inspires you. Now I'll show you how you can enjoy your vacation and not come home as big as a barge. Remember, losing weight is, to a large degree, a head game. With some simple rules in your head, you'll triumph.

Celebrate!

Most of us have reason to celebrate roughly once a week. Your birthday! Your anniversary! Your new job! Your new dress! Your newly mowed lawn! Yes . . . that's the plus and the problem: It's wonderful to have a life full of celebrations, but it's not so great when they involve food and become excuses to overindulge. So how do you let the good times roll while not adding to your roll? Here are my best strategies:

YOU SAY IT'S YOUR BIRTHDAY!   If it's a very special day for you, pick one meal—probably dinner—that you love and just enjoy it. You're a breakfast lover who craves pancakes? Go for it. Dessert is your temptation? Have a really special dessert and savor every bite. That doesn't mean turn the whole day into a binge, and you probably won't want to. But it's helpful to make a decision in advance on just how you're going to make your birthday special and then stick to that decision. What do you do about somebody else's birthday? Sometimes it's hard to know where to draw the line. I think it's best to do a cake taste only for immediate family—parents, kids, siblings, grandparents—and that's it! Enjoy a bite or two of the cake and count it as your carb for the day. Done.

Now or Never!

Many diets recommend that you should get started at some point in your life when nothing is going on so you can better control what you eat. Like when would that be? I say, *start right now*! You're *always* going to have things come up—special events and trips and holidays. If you put your life on hold for the sake of your diet, you're bound to fail. If you embrace your lifestyle and eat well in every situation, well, that's the key to permanent weight loss.

HAPPY HOLIDAYS   How long is a holiday? Some holidays can seem like they go on for weeks and weeks. (Ever hear of the twelve days of Christmas?) It can be a nonstop festival of cookies, fruitcake and special editions of M&M's and Hershey's Kisses. Obviously, a holiday that extends into a lifestyle isn't going to do your weight loss goals any favors. You don't want to be downing little candy hearts days after Valentine's Day nor shoveling mini Butterfingers in your mouth for the three weeks surrounding Halloween. Don't allow yourself to be swept into an extended celebration. Learn how to look at each in terms of a number of meals; for instance, decide that Christmas should be no more than about four festive meals. This will help you focus your energies on enjoying the special time without letting it derail you. Plan ahead and then work hard to stick with it.

HOME FOR A HOLIDAY   There's nothing better than being back in the nest for a special holiday. Well, maybe except for your hideously competitive sister-in-law. And your practical-joking brother. And how can any child whine so much? Oh well. They're family and you love them. Except when they try to force-feed you. Many of us fall into old familiar fourth-grade

Tips for Extended Holidays

Christmas, Hannukah Thanksgiving, Easter, Passover . . . how do you reign it in when everyone around you is eating nonstop? A few helpful suggestions:

✓ Start your day with a walk or run. If it's cold weather, bundle up and get out there and move. Do the twenty-minute rule: It's better than nothing and it will get your day off to a good start.

✓ Dress for success. In general, the more fitted your clothes, the less room you'll have to chow down. Guys, tighten that belt a notch or look for the slim-fitting shirts and slim jeans: You'll see a difference right away.

✓ Don't do a preparty starve. If you starve yourself all day in preparation for the big event it almost always backfires. It's just too hard to control yourself when you're crazy hungry.

✓ Sip seltzer. Use breath strips. Whatever it takes to keep food out of your mouth.

✓ Drink your water. Especially before a party. In the rush of the season, especially if you're traveling or visiting relatives, you can easily forget. Shoot for your four glasses by lunch. Even if you're making good food choices, holiday food is usually saltier and richer than normal and the water helps your body deal with the sodium so you don't bloat.

✓ Don't pick! One of the biggest challenges to maintaining your weight during holidays is snacking, so watch the bites, picks, and tastes. There's food everywhere, but don't allow mindless indulgences. Try to eat only at mealtimes. Keep the following in mind: One thumb-size piece of cheese costs you 100 calories, which takes about a mile of walking or running to burn off. That's just one little piece! The three examples below, easily consumed on a stroll through a holiday kitchen, add up to 200 calories or a two-mile walk or run. Think before you pick and taste!

» two spoons of chocolate chip cookie dough = 64 calories, 3 grams of fat

» leftover pie scraps = 81 calories, 5 grams of fat

» whipped cream licked off the beaters = 52 calories, 5 grams of fat

✓ Avoid the "ands." You know what I mean. Christmas dinner might be turkey. And stuffing. And green bean casserole. And potato. Pick the turkey and a couple of vegetables and just one starch (your mom's stuffing?). Then call a halt. You don't even really like Aunt El's sweet potatoes anyhow, do you?

patterns when we're back at home. Often our relatives encourage this. Many moms are never so happy as when they can feed you, and if they don't get to do it often, they want to make up for lost time. I tell my clients that how they handle this situation depends on their family dynamics. Some people find that it's best to call in advance and have a chat with Mom (or Dad if he's the chef) about your healthy goals and enlist their help. Maybe request a few more veggies and a little less lasagna. If you know that will go over like lead cannoli in your house, then you'll have to employ the stealth method of fake eating, where you push things around on your plate. I think one of the best antidotes to homecoming lethargy is to get moving. Plan some activities that the whole family will enjoy, whether it's a hike or a game of Wii tennis in the living room. (Just be sure to pick something that allows you to beat your sister-in-law.) If you can't get the whole family on the move, set your phone to work as an alarm and get out there early by yourself. A run or a brisk walk can really help put you in a good mental frame of mind for the whole day.

PROFESSIONAL PARTIES Many of my clients complain that their workplace is a nonstop festival. Birthday after birthday. Girl Scout cookie delivery day. TGIF, week after week. And then there are the out-of-office parties. It's a challenge to stick to a plan when every time you turn around someone is shoving a cupcake or piece of pizza your way. Here are some tips.

Office parties can be confusing because they pretend to be social events, but there is, or should be, a more formal undercurrent. You definitely don't want to cut loose the way you did at your best friend's wedding that resulted in all those embarrassing Facebook photos. So remind yourself that when you are attending a professional event the food is secondary to the connections and the business at hand. I always tell my clients to indulge with those you love. Never allow yourself to indulge at any business party. It's just never worth the calories. Office birthday and pizza-type parties are best battled with a strategic snack. You know if you're starving at 4 P.M. there's no way you're going to skip that cupcake or pizza wedge, so have your afternoon snack right before the gathering. Grab a water bottle from your office and smile, smile, smile. If you're sipping from your bottle and keeping your hands busy by helping serve, no one will notice that you skipped the goodies. If anyone asks, just say you had a late lunch and couldn't eat another thing. If the social dynamics of your work environment pressure you to partake, have a small amount of what's being served and push it around on your plate. People are typically so busy at a party that they're unlikely to notice you're not eating.

Don't Be a Hermit

Overwhelmed by the thought of dealing with gatherings when you're trying to lose weight? Some people think it's best to just lay low when they first go on a diet, avoiding every party, dinner and office event. This is not a good approach. For one thing, you know you feel guilty when you don't show up and this negative feeling can lead you to a pity party at home alone. It's also a Plunge waiting to happen when you begin to think about the opportunities you're missing to make social and work connections. It's important to learn to eat in the real world, in every situation. Rely on the Blueprint, banish your Devils and this time you'll keep the weight off forever.

Cocktail Parties, Buffets and Dinner Parties

Whether it's a holiday party, a gathering to celebrate your dad's retirement or your best friend's baby shower, parties always involve food and drink and require a little mental as well as physical prep if you want to enjoy the event and exit with your resolutions intact. Here are my top tips:

DRESS FOR SUCCESS When you look good you feel good, so ladies, take the extra time to treat yourself to a manicure, a hair appointment—even if it's just a roots touch-up—and pull that LBD out of the back of the closet. (If you don't have one, go get one!) Guys, a fresh shave, a haircut or a new shirt all contribute to a great party for you too. Feeling fabulous starts with dressing the part, and when you arrive at an event looking your super best you want to work the room and not the buffet table.

THE SLIMMING SNACK Never arrive at a social event ravenous. You know you won't be able to resist the crab dip and the cheese puffs if all you can think about is how starving you are. So enjoy a healthy snack about an hour or two before your event. Aim for something with 150 calories or less such as a Gnu bar or two FiberRich crackers with a Laughing Cow light cheese wedge. If you plan to drink, it also helps to have a little something in your stomach, so the alcohol won't hit you like a bomb.

KNOW BEFORE YOU GO If you know that there will be food at the party (and what gathering doesn't include food?), then decide in advance if the offerings will constitute your dinner. If yes, stick to the "four-napkin rule": Fill up three to four napkins' worth of appetizers in the course of the party and then stop! Go for the protein offerings that aren't fried such as shrimp cocktail, sushi, asparagus wrapped in prosciutto or chicken satay. No nibbling when you get home. If you're starving, you can have some turkey or hard-boiled egg whites. Remember that whatever four-napkins' worth of protein you choose counts as a carb. If you're not going to count the party as your dinner, have a plan in place. Get your snack and have plenty of water before the party. Have only one napkin's worth of protein if the hostess or anyone else pays attention. Make sure you have a dinner plan in place: I think the best bet is a frozen dinner. Skip any extra salad or veggies at home since you want to keep the volume low: It's probably later than your usual dinner. If you do go out for dinner after the party, go for the double appetizers or a very lean order. Check Dine-Out Devils (page 214) for Lean Order suggestions. Go to bed!

DELAY, DELAY, DELAY Try to delay both drinking and eating. Start with water or seltzer and make that work for you for a while. This gives you less time to overdo it, and you'll feel proud of your restraint (which will reinforce your good intentions). If the party includes a buffet or a sit-down dinner and you manage to avoid the hors d'oeuvres, you'll have that much more flexibility with your dinner choices.

CHAT IT UP   Sometimes we get so overwhelmed by party nerves that we forget why we're even out there, all dressed up. This can prompt nervous nibbling. Well, it's all about the meet and greet! Even if you're at a work event, it's great to take the opportunity to relax and enjoy the crowd. Meet some new people. Make some connections. If you decide that making friends is your goal, it's easier to focus on the people and not the peanuts.

BETTER BUFFETS   Buffets are a challenge. When you're trying to lose weight, confronting a buffet is the ultimate challenge. It's usually mountains of unlimited food. That's why you have to be mentally prepared and stick to the buffet rules, which are few and simple:

1. **STROLL THE LINE.** Check out all of the buffet foods, beginning to end. Normally the less expensive foods are right there in the beginning. You want to avoid the pasta salad and bread and wait until you reach the grilled meat or fish that are typically near the end of the table.

2. **YOU'RE NOT #1!** Don't be first in line. It's always hard to fight that urge, but it's much better to wait. While others are rushing back for mindless seconds, you'll be savoring your carefully curated plate.

3. **KILL THE CARBS.** You want to have a plate that's largely greens—vegetables of some kind—and lean protein. It's just better to avoid the carbs entirely, especially if you're having a drink.

4. **SKIP DESSERT.** It's just waaay too tempting to walk past a table groaning with brownies, cakes, cookies and

other sweets. So plan to skip entirely. If you see that there's fruit on the dessert table, you can serve yourself or even ask a friend to fill a plate for you. Enjoy your coffee or tea and there, you survived the buffet!

DINNER PARTY DILEMMAS   Dinner parties can be tricky when you're working hard to lose weight. It's so hard to be on the first week of your diet and get invited to a dinner party where the specialty of the evening is lasagna. But no one wants to have a guest who has a long list of food dos and don'ts. My basic advice for such situations (and this applies to both work and personal dining occasions) is if it's rude to refuse, just eat it. You don't have to finish every bite; in fact, try to leave about a quarter of it on your plate. And don't be tempted by the bread-basket or the dessert cookies since no one will notice that you're skipping those. What do you do when Aunt Ruth hands you the slice of pie that she made just especially for you—the one that required a special trip to a market two towns over so you could enjoy that pie you loved when you were five? Just eat it! Same with a business dinner where the boss insists that everyone enjoy his favorite dessert at his favorite restaurant. You don't always have to eat the whole thing. But it's much better to just smile and say thanks, as you reach for that slab of sugared fat than to make a fuss about how you can't eat things with a high glycemic index, blah, blah, blah. Once it's in front of you, you can simply ignore it: Chances are no one will notice.

Universal Party Rules

➤ Fitted outfit

➤ Strategic snack one hour before you head out

➤ Water, water, water before and during the party

➤ Breath strip before you make your entrance

MANAGE FOOD GIFTS   Gifts are often a part of celebrations, but food gifts can be the Trojan horses of your diet. You need ironclad strategies to deal with food gifts. You can't pause to consider what you're going to do with them because you know what that will lead to! First, if someone has baked something special for you and you're under immediate pressure (they're standing in front of you, wide-eyed, waiting for you to smack your lips!), take a small taste. Ohh and ahhh and then proceed to the next step: Give it away! You must have a neighbor, maybe an elderly friend, who would love to take it off your hands. How about the reception desk at work? The teachers' lounge at school? If worse comes to worst, into the trash it goes! One of my clients tells me that she forces herself to throw out food gifts and then immediately puts coffee grounds on them. Because, well . . . just in case.

Vacations and Their Devils!

Vacations should be enjoyed. They're interludes in our life that are truly special, and I think you should relax and enjoy your time away from the cares of regular life. Besides, a vacation usually lasts two weeks at the longest and you're ordinarily so busy—physically and mentally—that even if you're relishing new restaurants you're not going to gain that much. So don't be counting cheese tidbits and blanching at the thought of sauce on your grilled fish. At the same time, a few pointers will help you savor your meals while not losing control.

CONSIDER THE VACATION BONUS   Don't be afraid of your vacation. It will not ruin your diet. Many of my clients have been surprised to find that they can eat well on vacation without feeling restricted. And come home without gaining an ounce. For one thing, you aren't stressed on vacation. You may sleep

> ## Flying
>
> Is a flight in your future? If you're traveling by plane, I have just what you need to know to find healthy, satisfying food at the airport. Also, see RoadHogging, page 195, for tips that will help you get your vacation off to a great start.

better than at home. You are often exercising more: walking all day, swimming, skiing, climbing mountains. And you usually can't snack during the day! No wandering into the kitchen for a handful of raisins or dipping into the candy dish on the receptionist's desk. You're not cooking; you're not picking off the kids' plates. Take advantage of every pleasure of your trip, make sensible choices and you'll come home happy, relaxed and in the right frame of mind to lose even more weight.

GET OFF ON THE RIGHT FOOD   Don't you find that if you have a bad (food) beginning to a trip, things can go downhill? If you binge at the airport and you're busting out of your bathing suit on the first day, it sends you right to a caftan and the food bar. Feeling fat in the morning is depressing, and that's not how you want to feel on vacation. Have a good game plan for your departure day. Are you the type who thinks, "Whoopee! I'm on vacation! All the food is free!!" from the minute you lock your front door? Or, alternatively, do you get so stressed and nervous about travel of any type that you're searching for a comforting snack to calm your nerves hours before you approach your destination? I believe that mastering the first twenty-four hours of your vacation is the most important step you can take to maintain your weight loss goals. If you're heading to the airport, don't give in to the temptation to have a pastry or greasy slice of pizza because the fatigue and annoyances of travel make you want to self-medicate! If you like plane food and any is offered, don't be ashamed—just eat it. Try to skip the dessert if you can. And refuse those pretzels! They are wasted, salty calories. If you're traveling by car, pack healthy snacks and check in advance to find healthy meals en route. Check out RoadHogging, page 195, for specific tips about healthy eating while flying and driving. But remember, the most important thing is to get in a healthy mind-set right at the outset of your vacation: You're going to have a great time but you're going to make healthy choices. By the end of your vacation you're going to feel relaxed and slim and terrific.

SHOULD YOU SNACK PACK?   Although you shouldn't be a slave to your eating plan while on vacation, it's always wise to consider whether packing some snacks would be helpful. Are you going to a destination where healthy food might be a challenge? Are you the type of eater who can have snacks in your luggage but not binge on them at night? Will you be staying in a place with your own kitchen? In those cases, packing some bars and fiber crackers could be a wise move. But if you know you're going to have plenty of great food to sample or you have a tendency to abuse those snacks in your luggage, leave them home.

Basic Vacation Food Guidelines

Here are the modifications to the Blueprint that I suggest to everybody going on vacation. It's Blueprint Lite, with more flexibility and more fun.

1. Fat is free. Vacation is not the time to stress about sauce, condiments, cheese, eggs or red meat. Most of us are only on vacation for no more than a week, so the

little extra fat you might consume will be fine. It's one less thing to stress about when ordering, particularly if the menu is not in English. Of course if there are healthy options on the menu that you enjoy, choose them.

2. You can select one extra carb daily above your normal amount. When traveling outside the U.S. you can count a sandwich on white bread or pasta or rice as a carb.

3. Never choose a carb at breakfast.

4. One of your carbs, preferably your dinner carb, can be an indulgence such as a specialty food of the region.

5. Alcohol is free on vacation if it's wine, light beer, or vodka or scotch on the rocks or with club soda.

6. If you bring along snacks, never eat them after dinner; only eat them at snack time.

STAY STRONG AT BREAKFAST   Get your vacation days off to a good start by eating well at breakfast; it's well worth the effort. Whether you're at Disney World or in Fiji, you'll be able to find good options. There will be more temptations later, and a healthy, filling low-cal breakfast can be found no matter where you are. Don't waste your carb in the morning. First pause

Do Not Travel with Two Sets of Clothes

I've had clients who tell me that they bring along a "fat" and a "slim" wardrobe. This just sets you up for failure. Leave your baggy clothes home. While I don't think you need to focus on losing weight on vacation, it's really not that hard to maintain your weight.

and assess how hungry you are. Sometimes you'll still be full from the night before and can get by with a light breakfast or just some fruit and coffee or tea. But don't do this if you know it will make you so hungry that you'll lose control at lunch. If possible, try to order off the menu rather than be tempted by a breakfast buffet. But even if there's only a buffet, you can do a walk by and make healthy choices, and as you leave, grab an apple for a morning or afternoon snack.

Good buffet choices include:

➤ Any yogurt with high-fiber cereal (All Bran, Fiber One, Cheerios—avoid the granola) and fruit

➤ Two eggs (poached or hard-boiled are best) plus sliced tomatoes and fruit

➤ Egg white omelet (with veggies) and fruit

➤ If you're having a very hungry morning, you can add just one slice of either Canadian bacon or regular bacon. Skip sausage, since it's salty and not lean. Always skip the toast and any other carbs.

THE HAPPY HOUSEGUEST Sometimes you'll be spending part or all of your vacation at a friend or family's home. The most important thing to remember as a houseguest is not to pick between meals. Avoid the extra bowl of nuts or candies that adds up to too many calories. And sometimes when you're a houseguest there may be some level of social anxiety that prompts you to nibble. If you know your hosts well enough, it could be appropriate to mention that you're trying to eat well and ask if you can pick up a few things at the market. And this of course does not mean that you should entirely restock the fridge and pantry! Just be sure there's a good breakfast choice like low- or nonfat yogurt, some fruit and perhaps some sliced turkey and whole wheat bread for sandwiches. In general, it's more appropriate to just go with whatever is served for dinner, perhaps eating a smaller amount if it's something very rich. Of course there are also occasions when it's more of a work situation and you don't know the hosts well. In that case it's not appropriate to make any special requests. Just stick to your three meals and pay careful attention to your portions. Serve yourself less at meals, or leave a quarter of the food on your plate.

CHOOSE YOUR INDULGENCE   By now it's clear you shouldn't feel like you're in a food straightjacket while on vacation. With that in mind, you can choose one indulgence daily. Select the food indulgences that will really matter to you. If you're in Italy, you probably should be enjoying the pasta. You may want to try some fabulous hot chocolate in Paris. Don't say no to an evening of tapas in Barcelona. Decide what's going to give you the most pleasure and go for it. Just balance it out with healthy, lighter meals when you can. And it's usually wise to time your indulgence: One at dinner is usually safer than at lunch, which could set you off and make it harder to choose well for the rest of the day.

MOVE!   Most people find that they're naturally more active while on vacation. They're walking around as they sightsee, they're swimming, hiking, snorkeling, skiing and generally doing things that keep them in motion and burn calories. If your vacation tends to the sedentary, make a point to include some active time every day, whether it's a long walk or a stint at the hotel gym.

CLEAR THE MINIBAR   Never, ever, open the minibar in a hotel room unless it is to check that you don't get charged for a missing item. But beware the temptation to reach in for a bag of M&M's at midnight.

All Inclusive, Totally Abusive!

You know what I'm talking about: Those trips or cruises that are all inclusive when it comes to food. This often translates into a full-on binge as you take advantage of all the "free" food. People, step away from the buffet! While you want to enjoy your vacation, what's the point of overindulging just because it's "free"? Enjoy your food. Choose wisely. Eat well. Come home strong. You'll enjoy your vacation more.

WEIGH-INS ON THE ROAD?   Should you keep track of your weight while traveling? I actually had a client once who told me that a nutritionist had told her to carry a scale along with her while on vacation. This truly is ridiculous. For one thing, as I've mentioned, vacation is a time to relax. Your goal is not to lose weight but to maintain it. For most people their clothes will tell them if they're doing ok. Your clothes don't lie: If your pants are tight, you're going over the edge. If being out of touch with your weight gain or loss makes you anxious, then pack a soft tape measure. Check your waist measurement the day before you leave and every few days while traveling to see how you're doing.

REMEMBER RECOVERY?   Did you really overdo it at that fabulous restaurant in Trieste? Did you turn into a cordless Hooverer at that breakfast buffet? It happens. You're on vacation having a blast and then suddenly your clothes are supertight and you feel just gross. Solution? A Protein Day. Grab two poached eggs for breakfast, grilled chicken and salad for lunch and a small protein (steak, chicken, fish), salad and steamed veggies for dinner. By the next morning you'll be back on track.

SUMMER VACATION Some of us are lucky enough to have long stretches of vacation—for the luckiest it's Memorial Day to Labor Day—but for the rest of us there are at least long summer weekends. The downside to this blissful stretch of warm-weather free time is that it can be a huge struggle to stay on track. People assume it's easy to lose weight in the summer, but that's not necessarily true. Many of my clients say that they tend to gain more weight over the summer than any other time. There are beach days with lots of snacks, barbeques and outdoor parties. The solution is to decide that you're going to stay strong no matter what. For many people, the best summer goal is to simply maintain their weight and not gain.

➤ The most important segments of summer weekends are the bookends: As with any vacation start strong and end strong. On Friday night, pack a sandwich or have a game plan for where you can find a healthy meal. Have your return night plan in place: Know a good stop for a meal or stock your freezer so you'll have a tasty frozen dinner waiting.

➤ Stock your summer kitchen. Whether you're going to stay for a weekend or ten weeks, make sure you have plenty of healthy choices like yogurt, lots of fruits and veggies, healthy portion-controlled snacks, lean meats, chicken and fish. But don't be too restrictive or you'll find yourself ducking out for a giant soft-serve ice cream at the first opportunity. Allow yourself some treats so that you don't feel you're suffering.

➤ Take advantage of fresh produce to try new recipes. Summer offers a bounty of great, fresh, local fruits and veggies. Explore cooking sites like Epicurious.com to find fresh takes on old favorites—especially super-low-cal veggies like greens and squash.

➤ Get outside and move. Stick with your exercise routine. After all, you probably are more relaxed and have more time. But put more activity in your day: Go for a walk, a bike ride, a swim, play outside with the kids. You'll feel energized and it will keep you out of the kitchen.

➤ Pick from the best summer food selections:

- At a barbeque choose grilled chicken breast, salad, corn on the cob and roasted veggies.

- Best beach snacks include fresh or frozen fruit.

- Best alcoholic drink choices include vodka on the rocks with soda and lime.

➤ For lots more tips on summer survival strategies, see my blog at http://www.nu-train.com/blog.

RECOVER!   Your flight got in late. You're exhausted. Your in-box is full. You have ten thousand e-mails. The kids are a wreck. There's no food in the house and you're back to being chief cook and bottle washer: Reentry can be tough. You'd be surprised at how many of my clients master their vacation strategies, come home down a pound or two, and then begin shoveling in food the minute they're back in their nest. It's tempting to lose control and pig out. Don't! Recover instead with a Protein Day, a Volume Controlled Day or a Veggie Night. (See page 73 for details.) Choosing recovery instead of falling into a food abyss will help you readjust to civilian life and help ease your passage into everyday healthy eating. Remember vacation eating rules are only in play on vacation.

Diet Devil #9
Road Hogging

O n the road again. . . . How much time do you think you spend in your car each week? Ten hours? Six hours? Oh, baby . . . it's way worse than you think: The average American spends twenty-one hours a week strapped into their rolling second home, listening to the "recalculating" voice and wondering why traffic lights are not synchronized. Yes, indeed, many of us spend more time than we'd like en route. Driving the kids to and from activities. Commuting to work, running errands and, of course, taking those business trips that require planes, trains and automobiles. Getting from here to there as fast as you can is a fact of modern life. But something happens to us when we become bodies in motion. Is it the diesel fumes? The hum of the road? The cacophony in the back seat? ("Don't make me pull over!") Or is it simply that we want to be back home? There's nothing like traveling to transform you into a raving bottomless pit of indiscriminate cravings. Raise your hand if you've ever bought a Cinnabon at the airport or finished off two Happy Meals when your little ones changed their minds. And who doesn't know the greasy pleasure of devouring fast-food fries while driving? We've all been bedeviled by Road Hogging at one time or another.

Traveling can be stressful, inconvenient and tiring, so it's easy to forget all our good intentions while en route. And it can be hard to find healthy food on the road if you don't know what to look for. (America's favorite multitask: a drive-through restaurant!) Travel forces us off our schedules, throws monkey wrenches into our eating plans and generally disrupts our decision-making ability. Finally, many of us simply resent travel, even if unconsciously, and feel that we deserve a reward beyond watching the numbers on the odometer turn over or collecting airline miles for distance covered. And the best available reward may be a chocolate chip muffin and a mocha Frappuccino. But remember: Calories count, whether they're consumed in the air, on a train or from behind the wheel of a minivan. No matter how fast you're moving, the fat will find you.

The Road Hogging Devil is not the same as the food temptations you'll encounter during fun travel like vacations or holidays (see "Celebrations! Vacations!"). No, what I'm talking about here is the routine travel that includes everything from your daily commute to long road trips to business travel, all of which challenge your best-laid diet plans. And those early-morning trips in the dark to hockey practice or the long Friday drives to a weekend getaway or packing up the family for a visit to Grandma . . . they all count as times that you'll need some clever strategies to help you get over the hunger roadblocks.

There is an easy way to banish the Road Hogging Devil, and that is to simply *plan ahead*. It's amazing how often we just hop in the car or the taxi and take off, never thinking for a minute about where and what we might have for lunch and whether we're going to be desperate for something to eat in the next fifteen minutes. I think this is partly because there are so many food options everywhere—fast-food drive-throughs, diners, chain restaurants—that we never worry about filling our tummies. But the availability of countless food choices does not mean that all those options are good ones. Without a little advance thought and planning, too much travel time can encourage poor food choices and the overeating that packs on the pounds. On the plus side, fast food has become much, much healthier. For decades the top three chains specialized in burgers and fries. Now, two of the top three—Subway and Starbucks—offer calorie counts and healthy choices. So it's easier to eat well en route, but you have to know what you're doing.

What Road Hoggers Need to Know

Here are five effective strategies for those times when you look in the rearview mirror and a giant Road Hog is chasing you. They hold true whether you're riding in planes, trains or automobiles, for business or pleasure.

STAY STRONG   It's easy when you're on the road to make bad choices and simply write them off as "survival." ("I would never eat that at home." "I had no choice!") We've all done this. It's understandable, but really, you're only fooling yourself. So, whether you're hopping in the car for a day of family adventure or heading for the daily grind on your commute to work, have a game plan and visualize your day in advance: a healthy lunch stop? A good snack packed? A day, or part of a day, on the road shouldn't mean extra calories or extra volume. I love it when I see clients' food journals and I can't even tell that they've been on the road because their journals report the same healthy choices that they've been enjoying at home. So even while you're traveling try to keep your day as consistent as a day at home, meaning: breakfast, lunch, one snack and dinner.

SNACKS PACKS   Strategic snacking is one of the cornerstones of successful weight loss. And strategic snacking can prevent your trip—whether it's a long-planned business trip or a trip home for the holidays—from becoming a Devil Carb catastrophe. Pack some healthy snacks before you leave the house. If you're traveling with kids, you are probably used to stashing some snacks any time you hit the road. But make them healthy. Snacks will help you keep to regular mealtimes and will save you when you're miles from food but starving. And keep in mind: Try to stick with *the same eating schedule you follow at home.* The kids may need extra snacks, but you should try to limit yours to your normal routine, whether it's one afternoon snack or one mid-morning snack or both. It's tempting to munch away as you cover the miles, but just because the snacks are healthy doesn't mean they don't have calories and they don't count. (Five energy bars do not equal a healthy meal.) And of course the unhealthy ones are a disaster: The cookies, pretzels and animal crackers are not only high in calories, they leave you unsatisfied and eager for more! Some good on-the-road snack choices? How about Ziploc bags of raw veggies and cut-up fruit? Pack some FiberRich crackers and a few Laughing Cow light cheeses. Make sure you're also packing water. Energy bars are always handy. (See my recommendations for best bars on page 287) But always remember, "energy" means "calories"! The perfect mid-morning snack should be under 60 calories. A hand fruit or a string cheese are both fine. For your afternoon snack, choose a healthy bar that's under 180 calories and stick to just one bar. If you need an additional snack beyond your bar, stick to raw veggies (celery, cucumbers and peppers are great.)

DON'T BE FOOLED BY FATIGUE   Many trips include stretches of fatigue and we can often mistake fatigue for hunger. If you're feeling jetlagged, if your flight was delayed or if you arrive at your destination late, don't seek solace in carbs, no matter how strong your inclination. If you can't get in a quick workout to reset your clock, try a brief shower or a brisk walk around the neighborhood to get your bearings. Also, remember that dehydration can make you feel tired. In the frenzy of travel we can often skip our sips. Don't forget: Keep your water bottle handy.

STAY ACTIVE   It's tempting while traveling to convince yourself that just moving over the ground, in a plane, car, train or bus, counts as exercise. Unfortunately, you have to actually move your muscles. Whether you're on a car trip or a long flight, it's important to take stretch breaks. Get out of your seat and walk the aisle of the plane. Head to the galley in the back and do some stretches. If you're driving, break up the trip: Stop the car and go for a quick walk. Look for hotels that have fitness centers (most do these days). If you have a family at home, it can often be difficult to find time to exercise, but travel can actually create an *opportunity* for you. No dog to walk; no dinner to cook; no homework to supervise! Pack your sneakers and workout clothes. Don't make the excuse that "it takes up too much room": it's only sneakers, shorts, a top and a sports bra (for girls), and you can rinse them in the shower. If you are a runner, check the weather online at your destination so you can pack appropriate clothes for outdoor exercise. Get up a little early and squeeze in a workout, even if it's just twenty quick minutes on the treadmill; you'll get a terrific head start to your day. Exercise is a great way to smooth out the bumps in any road and make you feel more settled and in control.

BROWN BAG IS BEST   If you're traveling by car, bus or train it's easy to bring along your own food. When you pack it yourself, you can control your food and sidestep roadside calorie disasters. Brown bagging makes it easier for you to stick to your regular eating schedule: The food is ready when you are. This also prevents the delayed meals that can erode your determination to eat well. For breakfast you can take along two hard-boiled eggs or a high-fiber energy bar (Gnu or Oskri Fiber) or even an organic shake (Orgain is a good brand. It's an organic, ready-to-drink meal replacement that comes in some nice flavors). Then all you need is a hand fruit. For lunch or dinner a perfect choice is a healthy sandwich—turkey on whole wheat with mustard and lettuce is great; peanut butter and jelly for vegetarians—and a piece of fruit. Don't forget a few bottles of water.

Ok, you say brown bagging is just sooo . . . ugh! Here's how to make it more fashionable. I like these two good options for adult ecofriendly lunch boxes. So don't think of it as brown bagging; think of it as styling an earth-friendly, healthy meal! Try madebyoots (http://www.madebyoots.com/lunchbox.html). It's smart looking and helps with portion control, as well as lunch protection. And here's a "lunch purse" that will disguise your lunch as a stylish handbag, the best in stealth office brown bagging: http://www.lunchville.com/cgibin/commerce.cgi?search=action& keywords=lb100&template=PDGCommTemplates/TopBotNav/ SearchResult.html. Healthy lunches do not need to remind you of your third-grade lunchroom!

BEST BREAKFAST BARS   When you're traveling—driving, flying or just on your daily commute on a bus or train—it's useful to be able to toss a bar or two into your purse or briefcase to enjoy as breakfast. I've sampled countless energy bars and so have my clients; here are the ones that come out tops. The criteria I use for breakfast bars is that first, they can't have any chocolate. Chocolate first thing in the morning is a bad idea. It can really set you off on a sweets craving. The other criterion is lots of fiber. Most of us don't get nearly enough fiber, but my top breakfast bars really pack it on.

Need a Breakfast on the Fly?

Here are some of my top picks at popular spots. They may not be the healthiest low-cal breakfasts in the world, but they're good options when you need something en route. Keep in mind that if you're having a wrap or English muffin or flatbread at breakfast, it counts as a carb.

Starbucks

Perfect Oatmeal	140 calories without additions
Egg white spinach feta wrap	280 calories
Greek yogurt honey parfait	300 calories

Dunkin' Donuts

Egg white Turkey Sausage Wakeup Wrap	150 calories
Ham, Egg Cheese Wakeup Wrap	200 calories
Egg white Veggie Flatbread	280 calories
Ham & Cheese Flatbread	310 calories

Subway

Egg White Muffin Melt	140 calories

McDonald's

Egg McMuffin	300 calories
Yogurt Parfait	160 calories

➤ Gnu bar: At 130–140 calories the Gnu bar packs in half your daily fiber requirement. Even my male clients like Gnu.

➤ Oskri Fiber Bar: Oskri provides half your daily fiber at 150 calories.

➤ Cascadian Farm Almond Butter Granola Bar: A great choice if you like to crumble your bar into yogurt. 180 calories.

HYDRATE Many of us are reluctant to hydrate while on the road. Why? Because once upon a time we had to use a restroom at a gas station that looked like, well, let's just say it was truly unforgettable. But, really, isn't it time we got over that and recognized that there is no shortage of clean, functioning toilets? In fact, you can use SitOrSquat.com—a free app for the iPhone, iPod Touch and BlackBerry—which gives you the locations of over 105,000 (and counting) toilets around the world. Of course, there are also countless chain restaurants, coffee shops, stores and even roadside rest stops that you can easily find. Keeping up with your fluids really helps your digestion, which can become sluggish when you travel. We know that plenty of fluids give your metabolism the boost it needs to keep firing along at a nice calorie-burning rate. It also keeps your immune system strong. While travel can take a toll, with lack of sleep, cramped spaces, free-range germs on trains and planes, extra water will keep your defenses operating at peak performance. Of course the great big RoadHogging reason to hydrate is that it keeps you feeling full and less likely to overeat. So pack your water bottle and sip regularly.

TRANSFORM BUSINESS TRAVEL If you do a lot of traveling for business you often endure a host of conditions that prompt you to abandon all your healthy resolutions. You're tired, you're stressed, and yes, you're often resentful because you've had to leave your family and friends and comfy bed behind. I always tell clients that the time to indulge is when they're with friends and family, not in a work situation. That holds doubly true with business travel. Though you may be tempted to indulge to reward yourself for your hard work, it's so much better to save those indulgences for when you're back home with those you love. So, while many of my clients complain that business trips are the death of their diets, it doesn't need to be this way. Try to look on the bright side: You're free of daily chores, you're often staying at nice hotels, you can hop out of bed and be on your way—no walking the dog, loading the dishwasher, chasing the kids. . . . So try to get into a "spa" mind-set while on the road. Take advantage of downtime to exercise. Make a point of choosing light, healthy meals, and be determined to come home a few pounds lighter. You'll enjoy an indulgence or two when the long and winding road is behind you.

These strategies will help all travelers stick to their diet resolutions. But there are other speed bumps along the road that can make resolutions evaporate. Let's take a look at the three most common Road Hogging Devils and how to survive them:

➤ Road trips

➤ Air travel

➤ The commute

Road Trips

The advantage of road trips is that you have greater control over what you eat because you can turn your vehicle into a healthy food source. That's right: Nothing's stopping you from filling a cooler with healthy snacks, some wonderful healthy sandwiches and a few water bottles.

Of course sometimes you have to be on the road beyond the distance your packed food can take you. And then you will be prey to the fast-food establishment. Actually, there are healthy choices to be had at almost all fast-food chains these days. But you have to know how to navigate the drive-through because there are surprises: At McDonald's, for example, the plain burger is 250 calories while the Southwest crispy chicken salad is 430 calories. At Burger King the burger is 260 calories and the chicken club is 630 calories! Obviously, at McDonald's you're better off having a plain burger than the crispy chicken salad. I have done all the work of picking out the best fast-food choices and you'll see them on page 261. If you're headed on the road soon, take a minute now to scan the fast-food lists and jot down your top choices at any of the fast-food chains that you're likely to visit. Stick your list in your purse or glove compartment. There: You're road ready!

I know that when you're out on the blue ribbon of highway, fast-food options are overwhelmingly popular and the food court can be an easy solution, especially if you follow my suggestions for good choices at fast-food places as listed below. The best approach is to check online for the calorie counts of foods at the chain restaurants you tend to visit. Try to find selections that are between 300 and 400 calories for lunch or dinner (lower for women; higher for men). In general, I find the healthiest food options are at Subway, Cosi, Quiznos and Starbucks. Subway, in particular, is usually very easy to find and offers a line of healthy meals called Subway Fresh Fit Meals, which include a sandwich, a fruit and a bottle of water. A veggie or turkey sandwich on this meal is between 200 and 300 calories, which is a great calorie count for a very satisfying lunch. And there's something about having a good-sized sandwich for lunch that makes you feel happy and satisfied and doesn't scream, "Oh, poor me, I'm on a diet but I have to watch everyone eat a big fat burger and a funnel of fries." Ask them to toast the bread on your Subway sandwich; it boosts the flavor nicely. And skip the cheese.

Air Travel

Ah yes, the airport, where good resolutions go to die. Airline travel is surely the most trying to those of us struggling to eat healthy foods and stick to our resolutions. Flying these days is typically a stress festival. From the moment you leave your house—often at a hideously early hour—to the moment you deplane—often past your expected arrival—the assaults on your serenity are too numerous to name. But just to list a few, there's the getting up in the dark, the wait in endless lines with other cranky people, the virtual strip for strangers and the wedging yourself into a tiny seat in a metal tube that's supposed to go up in the air and then get down again safely (How, I ask you? How?). And there's almost no food. And let's not forget that the food that you do encounter in the terminal is, well, just about terminal: Cinnabons, Sabrett's pizza, giant muffins and so on, all washed in the scent of diesel fuel. Plus you're tired and you wish you were home. It's a definite diet challenge. But you can do it! Here are my never-fail air travel tips:

BEFORE YOU GO   The day before you head out the door, make a trip to the grocery store and pick up a couple of healthy frozen dinners. When you get home from your travels and you're tired and hungry and considering a big, comforting carryout order of General Tsao's chicken, you can, instead, pop your healthy frozen meal into the micro, relax with a simple dinner, and get right back on your healthy track. See my suggestions for postflight frozen meals (page 285).

STICK TO YOUR PLAN   Air travel is particularly disorienting. You're on a different schedule and you're at the mercy of the weather and you often feel entirely out of control. Don't let that general sense of disorder spill over into your eating plans; as much as possible, try to stick to your basic at-home eating routine. Eat your three meals, enjoy your snacks (if any) and make wise choices. Once you skip meals or start mindlessly nibbling, you begin to lose control. Don't tell yourself, "I'm just going to snack." (Those trail mixes are filled with a day's worth of calories!) Find a real, healthy meal and avoid the bits of this 'n' that. Even if the only meal you can find is not at the pinnacle of best diet choices, it's still better than unsatisfied snacking. If you eat a real meal, you'll feel better and you'll arrive at your destination with the confidence of being in control.

BRING YOUR OWN?   I don't think it's worth it to fuss too much about bringing food along to the airport. You really can find most anything you'd need there. You're usually in such a rush that there's not much time for food prep before you head out any-way. One suggestion, however, that my clients swear by: Bring along your own fiber crackers—either GG Bran Crispbreads or FiberRich Bran Crackers. They are the Swiss army knives of snacks. They can help fill you up if a meal or flight gets delayed, they can be crumbled into yogurt to add some crunch to your breakfast, they can give you something to nosh on if you need a snack at any point in your trip. If you like, toss in a Laughing Cow light cheese in any flavor (they now come in blue cheese as well as creamy garlic, among others) in your bag. They don't need refrigeration and, smeared on a fiber cracker they make a great, filling snack. Just be sure to keep up with your water in-take to wash all that fiber down.

Many of my clients like to toss some packable healthy foods in their bags, especially if they're going to be away from home for a few days. These foods can serve as snacks or even as meal replacements if necessary. (See page 287 for more detailed suggestions on packable foods like energy bars.)

Packable Power Foods

➤ Instant oatmeal packet under 150 calories (see p 280 for brands)

➤ Kashi Go Lean individually packed cereal

➤ FiberRich crackers (2): 40 calories

➤ GG crackers (2): 24 calories

➤ Justin's nut butter packets (2 tbsp): 190 calories

➤ Barney Butter 100-calorie packet

➤ Emerald or Blue Diamond 100-calorie bags of raw almonds

➤ Mini Babybel Light cheese (1 round): 50 calories

➤ Laughing Cow cheese (does not need refrigeration): 35 calories

➤ Mini Cabot cheese (¾ oz bar; lactose free): 50 calories

WIN THE BREAKFAST BATTLE Breakfast really is important since it sets you up for a healthy day and gives you the nutrition you need to help you make good food choices at lunch. But when you're flying, you often have to leave your house at such an early hour that you become dependent on terminal offerings to get your food day started. And that's not always a pretty sight. Not to worry: I have easy solutions that have worked for me and for my clients. Skip the giant pillow bagels (although they could be useful as neck rests!) and pick either one of my sure-fire healthy, filling, über-available terminal breakfasts:

➤ Coffee shop instant breakfast: Any airport coffee shop—and there's always one open—can help you here.

Order a venti skim latte. Yes, indeed, a venti skim latte really can be the cornerstone of a healthy breakfast. It's a shot of espresso along with about 9 ounces of milk that adds up to about 200 calories. You can order it with skim or soy milk, and although the soymilk has a bit more sugar in it, it's still a good choice. Round out this breakfast with a piece of hand fruit like a banana. How easy was that? Is it the best breakfast choice in the world? Heck, no! But it's a nice dose of calcium, protein and even a few phytonutrients. And it will hold you for a few hours until lunch. And it's soooo much better than many of the other airport choices.

➤ Bigger instant breakfast: OK, so you have a few more minutes. Or you're extra hungry or you're a guy and really need more food than my coffee shop breakfast. Get your coffee or tea at Starbucks or any coffee shop. While you're there, pick up a non- or low-fat yogurt and a piece of fruit. Next stop is Hudson News, which you can find in almost any airport and which always seems to be open no matter how early. There you can find a good selection of energy bars. Pick up an energy bar (and maybe an extra one for a snack later on in the day, depending on the length of your trip,) and there's your bigger breakfast: coffee or tea, yogurt, fruit and an energy bar. You've got your protein, fiber, calcium and you're on your way!

Best Quick, Healthy Airport Food Picks

While breakfast seems to be the biggest airport challenge, you definitely will be looking for food at other times en route. You also might have to purchase a meal to carry aboard. (Keep

Super Flight Sites

Here are some excellent sites that can help make your trip less stressful and healthier:

✓ *Gate Guru* (gateguruapp.com): Detailed airport maps save you from going through security only to find the sole restaurant on the other side is a vending machine. Includes a simple search engine for foods, shops and services with ratings, reviews and photos.

✓ *Flight Board* (mobiata.com): Track every aspect of your flight, including delays, cancellations and gate changes for over 5,000 airports and 1,400 airlines.

✓ *Urbanspoon* (urbanspoon.com): Finding good and healthy places to eat can be a challenge but not when you rely on *Urbanspoon* to guide you. No matter how strange the city, this site can help you find addresses, reviews, directions and even help you make reservations at countless local eateries.

✓ *Airline Meals* (http://www.airlinemeals.net/index.php): Wondering what, if anything, they'll be serving on your flight? Check out this site. It's the world's largest and leading Web site all about flying food. It's a helpful, if sometimes scary (there are photos!) resource.

in mind that most airports allow you to bring food through security now with the exception of liquids, Jell-O, yogurts, etc. If you take medications, you can travel with water. Check with your airline in advance.) To help you make good choices at the airport, here are my suggestions:

➤ **SANDWICH:** Look for simple sandwiches on whole wheat bread. Try to find those with nutrition labels. Many places like Starbucks have calories listed on their sandwiches. Choose ones under 380 calories. Avoid sandwiches with mayo, bacon, tuna salad or egg salad and opt for a veggie sandwich or one with lean protein (turkey or chicken), of course without mayo. Added lettuce and tomato is fine.

➤ **SALADS:** Look for the grilled chicken Caesar; they are everywhere from fast-food spots to bars. Dressing always comes on the side when salads are made to go. balsamic vinaigrette is usually a good choice.

➤ **YOGURTS:** You can find these at any airport food stand. Pick Greek, low- or nonfat and reduced-sugar varieties. (Pack a small Ziploc of it with Fiber One or Kashi Go Lean cereal for extra crunch.) Skip most yogurt parfaits, since they tend to have high-sugar yogurt and granola mixed in, which sneaks in lots of extra calories. (Starbucks and McDonald's yogurt parfaits are the exception. The Starbucks version is made with Greek yogurt and is high in protein, and the McDonald's version is low in calories.)

➤ **FRUIT:** Look for the hand fruit. You'll always find an apple, orange or even small banana that you can literally grab as you run through the airport. Pair it with the yogurt and a granola bar and you've got a breakfast!

AWESOME AIRPORT FIND! CIBO EXPRESS GOURMET MARKET
Now located at Kennedy, LaGuardia, Philadelphia, Dulles, Logan, Reagan, Tucson International and Orlando Airports, this is the best place to grab a snack before you jet. The bar selection is great, and you'll find additional healthy options such as fresh fruit, Greek yogurt, vegetarian sandwiches (with the calories listed), hard-boiled eggs and more.

REENTRY You're back! You may be tired and cranky. Or you may be refreshed and filled with wonderful memories. Whatever the residue of your trip, it's important to ease back into real life with all your healthy resolutions intact. It's always a little disorienting to be home after travel, so keep things simple: Enjoy the frozen dinner you'd stashed before you left. Take a bath or shower. Get to bed on time. And, my best suggestion for the "party's over" blues: make your next day a Protein Day (see page 75). You'll recharge and get control and stay strong.

The Commute

If you commute to work, that daily morning and evening grind can take a toll on your diet. That's because you're forced into eating patterns that may not appeal to you and you typically don't have the time to enjoy a healthy, satisfying breakfast. Many of my clients get up very early in the morning to get to work. They tell me that they wolf something down before they leave the house but they barely taste it. Or they skip eating entirely and have a coffee on the bus or train or in the car. When they arrive at work they're starving and pressed for time, so they grab bacon, egg and cheese on a roll or perhaps a big bran muffin or maybe a bagel. These morning habits begin to take a toll on your waistline, since they're usually too high in calories and too low in protein to satisfy you until lunch. They also tend to be very high in carbs and thus can cause blood sugar spikes that make you desperate for that mid-morning coffee to fight off the postcarb slump.

There's no denying that breakfast is the most important meal of the day as far as weight loss goes. There's some evidence that it primes your metabolism to continue to burn calories at a good rate throughout the day. And if it's a healthy breakfast it will keep you satisfied so you won't be tempted by mid-morning snacks or a binge at lunch. So the first thing you need to decide if you commute is *when* you're going to enjoy your best healthy breakfast. The key concept here is a *single* breakfast. Those that grab something at home and then something else at work find it very difficult to shed weight. I think it's important to consider where you will have the time to actually taste and enjoy your food. If you're so rushed in the morning that you simply gulp down something at home and again at the office, then you need to carve out at least ten minutes—at one place or the other—to enjoy your meal. One of the problems with eating distractedly is that you don't really feel that you've eaten anything!

You often hear that you should be eating your breakfast shortly after waking. I have never seen research to back this up, and it's certainly not held true in my experience working with clients. Many of them delay breakfast until they get to work. They simply don't have the time to eat at home. They grab a coffee at home or on the way and eat something when they arrive at work. There's nothing wrong with this as long as you make good choices. If you are not hungry in the morning, have a coffee or tea or whatever your morning beverage is and head off to work. If you are hungry, eat a piece of fruit early and then save some additional breakfast—like yogurt—to enjoy once you arrive at work. Make your breakfast schedule work for you! See page 26 for healthy choices at chain restaurants because hopefully many of those same chains—like Starbucks or Dunkin' Donuts—will be located en route to your office.

If you have the luxury of being able to eat at home, take advantage of that. It should be easy for you to choose something healthy every morning. Most of my clients are Phase Eaters at breakfast: They repeat the same breakfast almost every day, usually on a seasonal basis. The most common healthy breakfast choices are Greek yogurt with fruit and some Kashi cereal for crunch in the summer and oatmeal with fruit in the winter.

A couple of hard-boiled eggs and some fiber crackers are another popular choice that has the advantage of being easy to eat on the run. Whatever you choose, take a few minutes to savor it as you get your day off to a healthy start.

And let's not forget about the commute home. The biggest danger with the return trip is finding yourself so hungry that you buy treats on the way or else you arrive home so hungry that you dive right into a bowl of cereal or something worse before a healthy dinner. Most commuters need an afternoon snack—something an hour or so before they leave the office—to keep hunger at bay. So keep something in your desk drawer. If you're challenged by hunger as you leave work, try saving your usual afternoon snack (that you might have at 3:00 or 4:00 P.M.) and enjoy it on the ride home. You might have a tea and a hand fruit in the office and then your 180-calorie snack (see the snack choices on page 286) for the return commute.

Diet Devil #10
The Dine-Out Devil

Wake up, America! You can't eat out (and that means takeout too) three, four, five times a week without gaining weight unless you have a strategy. Eating out is a huge and frighteningly powerful Diet Devil, because the simple fact is that restaurant food and fast food can make you fat. There are three easy ingredients that make food taste good: fat, salt, sugar. When you can't control your fat, salt and sugar intake, you're in trouble. There's also the psychological aspect to eating out: It feels like a mini vacation. Who wants to behave on vacation? So most people aren't in the mean-and-clean mind-set when they're sitting with friends with a lobster bib tied around their necks or facing a seven-course extravaganza with a chilled glass of champagne.

I didn't realize that eating out was a serious Devil until I first started working with clients in New York who were successful corporate types. Many of them told me that they'd first gained weight when they started entertaining for work. It seemed like a thrill to be able to try all the hot restaurants and to eat *for free* three or four nights a week. What could be more fun? But then their clothes got tight and the thrill of the porterhouse with the creamed spinach or the grilled cod cheeks with pureed fava beans began to pale. So the challenge was how to eat out constantly and not gain weight. And how do you do it while still enjoying a glass or two of wine with dinner? (Because almost every single client told me, "I will give up some things but I will not give up alcohol.")

You don't have to be a corporate titan to be vulnerable to the Dine-Out Devil. Anyone who's found himself at the fast-food drive-up window or who's left her book club dinner feeling like she would need to jog the Great Wall to work off her dinner knows it's just not easy to eat healthy when you're not in your own kitchen. There's the breadbasket, the group ordering, the "just-a-taste" desserts, the french fries for the table. . . . Don't despair! You can do it. You just need some clever strategies to help you deal with the devilish temptations of eating out. And the good news is that some restaurants are making the effort to help you: I just heard an advertisement for a high-end New York restaurant that's now offering smaller portions at smaller prices. Plus, you can now often find calorie counts at chain restaurants, which is a terrific—and sometimes eye-opening— help to those of us working to stay healthy. And finally, for some people, eating out can actually move them closer to their weight loss goals. If you choose wisely from the menu, learn to manage buffet offerings and avoid snacks at home, your food intake can be varied and controlled. Plus, there are no second helpings or midnight leftovers, no feelings of social isolation to push you into a binge!

How to Conquer the Dine-Out Devils

IT'S A MIND GAME Enjoying a healthy and satisfying meal in a restaurant, while you enjoy the company of friends, lovers or even business associates, begins in your head. It's important to remind yourself that eating in a restaurant isn't permission to abandon all your good intentions because it's free or it's tempting or because good fellowship encourages you to indulge. It's not always easy: You've got a warm breadbasket in front of you, a waiter eager for your drink order and a menu that lists a host of tempting selections. But try to think of eating out, or ordering in, as an opportunity to eat tasty, healthy food that you don't have to cook, instead of a vacation from your resolutions.

BREAD REALLY IS THE DEVIL   White, brown, seed, popover, sourdough . . . when it comes to dining out, they're all Devils. That damn breadbasket can't wait to get you. It's poppable, hot, infinitely refillable and it comes with killer sidekicks: butter and olive oil. And just when you thought you were safely at your appetizer, the bread guy returns with more hot, crusty tempting bread. For me and for most of my clients, bread in a basket is a trigger food—a trigger that can set you off on a diet-destroying meal. We are all used to blaming the salt, the fat, the oil and the portion sizes for the risks in dining out. But I've come to believe that the greater peril is the bread—and the fries, pasta and dessert that come avalanching down on us after the bread. I used to take the typical nutritionist route when I ate out: I'd deconstruct everything and eat a plain, simple, steamed, poached, totally boring meal. No fat; no flavor; no food in my food; no fun. And then I'd get home and hit the fridge. Or I wouldn't even make it home; I'd dive into a giant, compensatory dessert, scarfing up everything in the late-night bodega. I needed a new strategy. Here's my dine-out secret: Skip the breadbasket! Do whatever it takes. Sit on your hands; take a bathroom break, talk. . . . If you absolutely must, take a piece and play with it. Roll it into little balls. When it's time to order, you're already ahead of the game. You can enjoy some real food, prepared and served the way the chef thinks it should be served and, best of all, you'll be satisfied by all the terrific flavors. If you stick to some version of a salad and a grilled, sautéed or baked protein or veggie dish, you're going to enjoy your meal and be satisfied. You will have conquered the Bread Devil.

ADVANCE MENU ALERT As you good scouts know, planning ahead saves the day every time. This is especially true for making good choices in a restaurant. Haven't you sometimes found yourself settling in at a table with a group of people—some of whom you may have just met—only to feel like a deer in headlights when the waiter begins to take orders? You haven't had time to think about it; haven't stopped chatting long enough to study the options. Someone else says "fettuccine" and you say "me too." Don't let this happen to you. Take a minute to check the menu before entering the restaurant. Technology is your best friend these days, since you can simply log on to a host of Web sites—including the restaurant's—to read the menu and see what looks good and healthy to you. Handy online menu sources include *Menupages*, *Seamlessweb* and *Menutopia*. These sites have applications to download to your phone so that you can even check the menu en route. Pick two things in case they run out of your first choice.

BE A STEALTH DIETER You don't always want your dining companions to know that you're watching what you eat. This is especially true if you're eating out with business contacts, a first date or people you don't know well. You may have to just roll with it and do the best you can. Remember that it's best to be the last to order. By then, no one is paying attention to your choice. Keep in mind that you don't have to finish all the food on your plate: Eat half of what you're served. But even if you're with friends, you don't want to become that annoying person who deconstructs every dish, asking the waiter to "take out" this and "skim" that and put most everything else on the side. Try to limit yourself to one special request. Be strategic with your choices: Pick a salad with a vinaigrette dressing rather than a creamy one. Another simple and easy-to-manage request is, "Can I get double sautéed spinach, hold the risotto (or other starch), please?"

My Top Stealth Orders:

➤ Eggs Benedict with sauce on the side. You can enjoy the two poached eggs and half of the English muffin plus a piece of the Canadian bacon.

➤ Topless burger. Strip the top off that burger and load up on veggies. This is a great option for all those times that burgers are one of the few choices. A topless burger gives you some of the bread but half of the calories. And it's a Stealth Order!

➤ Grilled chicken Caesar with dressing on the side. You can request some oil and vinegar on the side. Eat around the croutons.

WATER YOURSELF   Ever notice how your face can sometimes look really puffy in the morning when you've eaten out the night before? You know—that two tiny eyeballs and two giant cheeks look? Or sometimes it doesn't show up in your face but rather on the scale: five pounds heavier in twenty-four hours! Well sodium can be a real issue when dining out, especially if you're not a good water drinker. Try to get in your eight cups of water before you have your dinner out to help your body handle the extra salt in the meal itself.

The Best Defense

Have you ever ordered a salad and had someone at the table make a snide comment about healthy eating? Sadly, there are sometimes frenemies or competitive people who may make you feel uncomfortable about your healthy choices. This situation puts a weird kind of pressure on you that can sometimes catapult you into a Plunge just to prove you're "one of the guys." Don't let the haters intimidate you. Here are some comebacks that can help:

> Q: "Have a dessert, for goodness sake. It won't kill you."
>
> A: "Yes, it will."
>
> Q: "Have another glass of wine. You a teetotaler or something?"
>
> A: "I've still got a buzz on from this morning."
>
> Q: "Why aren't you eating your potato?"
>
> A: "I saw the waiter lick it."

SNACK STRATEGICALLY   The last thing you ever want to do is arrive at a restaurant when you're totally, absolutely, insanely starving. You know what a recipe for disaster that can be! Bring on the bread! Appetizers all around! Full speed ahead! The best way to stay in control is to enjoy your afternoon snack one or two hours before you sit down at the restaurant. And if you don't routinely have an afternoon snack, it could make sense to have one on those days when you're eating out. Try two FiberRich crackers or an apple. The snack will take the edge off your appetite and help you make better choices. Water can help too. A glass or two of water within the hour before your restaurant date will also help make you feel full. (And don't forget to sip your water throughout the course of your meal. It will distract you from your food, help you to eat more slowly and also make you feel fuller.)

PUT ON THE BRAKES   A few little tricks in your back pocket are the ultimate eating-out fail-safe. The point of fine dining out is that it really tastes good, so slow down and taste it. Sip that water! Make sure to get your water glass filled up at least three times. It will also give you something else to do so you actually slow down. Another way to pump the brakes is to put down the knife and fork. You'll be surprised how difficult this is, as most of us cling to our utensils as some sort of shield and sword of dining, but it will help you slow down if you give them a rest now and again and join in the conversation. Remember, there's no prize for finishing first.

MANAGE ALCOHOL   Many of my clients flat-out refuse to eliminate alcohol from their diets. I completely understand. Some people are just not prepared to live the rest of their lives without alcohol, so I wanted to create an eating program that would work for them forever! It is possible to lose weight and drink

Fast Eater Survival Tip

All of us benefit from eating more slowly. But some people need extra help. I've had clients who can devour an entire meal before others can get through their appetizer. For those folks, I suggest "working food," that is to say, food that slows you down. So, for example, you might do better with a plate of mussels than a plate of scallops. You might consider ordering a filet of beef as opposed to a stew. A whole fish is an excellent choice. It's light and healthy and takes a long time to eat. Anything that is time consuming to eat will work to your advantage.

socially. But it's critical to manage alcohol consumption. We all know that drinking lowers your resistance, leading to Plunges. If you lose control of your eating when you drink, or if you lose control when you're hungover, then you definitely have to cut back on your drinking if you really want to lose weight.

Here's my basic rule of alcohol: One drink is free but the second drink counts as an Angel Carb. (You'll see in the Blueprint how many carbs you can have daily.) The best drink to choose is one you're not that crazy about. Why? So you'll drink slowly! For most people, especially women, simple drinks like vodka or scotch with soda are usually a good choice. Wine, especially white wine, goes down too quickly and easily. You'll also notice that waiters are quick to refill an empty wine glass. You have to order a refill on a mixed drink, thus giving you better control over your consumption. (If you're in a situation where the waiter tried to refill your drink, simply wave him away with a flip of your hand.) My own go-to drink is vodka soda with lemon or lime. Each sip of vodka is like a little pinch, reminding me to eat well. A light beer in a bottle is also a good choice: Beck's Premier Light is only 64 calories (skip the Sierra Nevada at 200 calories per bottle).

If everyone is having a cocktail before the meal, try to delay drinking for as long as you can. Have a club soda with lime—this looks enough like a mixed drink to fool people. And it allows you to delay your alcohol until dinner. If there's a toast, take a sip but don't suck down the whole drink. The goal is not to begin to drink (except for a toast) until the appetizer arrives. Many people finish their first drink before they even have a bite of food, and that's a bad idea because the effects of alcohol are magnified on an empty stomach. Make sure you have a glass of tap or mineral water at hand. No one will really notice that you're not drinking alcohol and that water will keep your hands busy and also fill your tummy.

Many of us forget that alcohol can pack a caloric wallop. Some drinks—particularly mixed drinks like margaritas and cosmos—are highly caloric. And there are other considerations: That brunch favorite—a Bloody Mary, for example—is loaded with salt. So while an 8 ounce Bloody Mary has about 140 calories it's the salt in the tomato mix that can do even more damage. If you're salt sensitive, a drink like this can increase your sugar cravings throughout the day. You may be proud you passed on the pancakes at brunch, but the cookies may be calling your name come mid-afternoon.

Alcoholic Drink Picks

Reminder! Since we agreed the first drink is on the house but the second one will count as one Angel Carb, I recommend choosing the drink that you can drink the slowest to make sure you take your time.

Alcohol Best Bets	Calories
Glass of red or white wine (6 oz)	140
Light beer (12 oz)	99
White wine spritzer	75
Vodka and soda (or diet tonic)	100
Scotch on the rocks	100

PERILS OF PORTIONS   You already know that reduced volume is critical to weight loss. What you may not know is my rule of Champagne Reduction: The more expensive the meal, the smaller and healthier the portions. On the other hand, the less expensive the meal, the more careful you have to be to guard against GIANT amounts of food that are higher in salt and fat than you'd like. Very high-end restaurants dazzle their clien-

Family-Style Group Orders

What could be more fun than a family or group of friends gathered at a restaurant to celebrate or to just have fun? Of course the problem is that you may not be in charge of ordering your own meal. The solution? First, check the menu in advance if you can so you'll be armed with a few good choices if you get the opportunity to put in your vote. Once you're at the restaurant, roll with the punches: The point is to have fun, not fuss. At the same time you should make your wishes known if possible. A key point is to avoid the bread, pasta, fries, fried food and desserts. Remember the sauces count as carbs. With each course, try to suggest something healthy: There's almost always a salad option at most any restaurant. For the entrée, suggest a grilled protein. And always suggest side veggies. When the food comes, no double dipping; only add food to your plate once and that includes veggies. Try to stay an arm's length from any desserts or biscotti that land on the table. Claim you're stuffed! Order some peppermint or chamomile tea to finish.

tele with fresh and exotic ingredients and exquisite preparation techniques as well as photo-ready presentation. Your local diner knows that a big yellow haystack of mac 'n' cheese is the way to please the crowd. Sometimes you just crave inexpensive comfort food. That may be OK, as long as you eat only about a quarter of what you're served. Don't fool yourself into thinking that two appetizers at a Ma and Pa eatery is going to equal in calories two appetizers at the latest star chef's hotspot. If you're going to hit up the neighborhood diner, try to share an entrée. And don't worry too much about asking for substitutions on the menu (e.g., greens instead of fries); you're probably not going to offend anyone. Or you can order only an

Hari Hachi Bu

The Okinawans embrace cultural portion control. They call it *hari hachi bu* and it is the practice of eating only until you feel about eighty percent full. Leaving twenty percent of your food behind is a good strategy to avoid obesity. And you won't go hungry because it takes you about twenty minutes to feel full from a meal and if you leave the table eighty percent full, in twenty minutes you'll feel completely full. On twenty percent less food!

appetizer. Just remember that it's so tempting to finish everything on your plate that you're going to have to practice some restraint.

ONE OUT OF THREE   The key to healthy dining out is to keep it simple. After all, the large number of choices is what prompts us to overeat. So here's another simple rule to bear in mind. It will guide you toward a healthy, low-cal, low-volume meal. When eating out or ordering in, skip the bread, skip the dessert and choose *just one* out of three possible indulgences:

➤ One extra alcoholic drink (remember, the first drink is always free)

➤ Yummy sauce on your dish (doesn't count if it's just a bit of olive oil)

➤ A fist-sized Angel Carb (baked or roasted potato, rice, quinoa, farro, etc.)

If you decide in advance to follow the one-out-of-three rule, you'll be able to clear your head of all the possible temptations and you'll feel in control.

SATISFYING MINI ORDERS   You don't always have to order an appetizer, an entrée and a dessert. Now you undoubtedly knew that but it's worth the reminder. I tell clients there are three ways to order healthy:

➤ Two appetizers and a side veggie

➤ An appetizer and an entrée

➤ Just an entrée

If you're ordering, say, two appetizers and a side veggie, tell the waiter when you'd like them served. The idea is to be eating with the group. So you might have one appetizer when others are enjoying their appetizer and the other app and the veggie while the others have their entrée. The key here is to know yourself: if two appetizers are going to leave you hungry and reaching for the breadbasket, then it's best for you to stick to an entrée.

LUNCH TIPS   If you're having a restaurant lunch in the middle of your workday, keep it clean. Lunchtime orders should always be lower fat and lighter than a dinner meal. Consider double appetizers, hold sauces, go very light on the fats. Choose fish, even if you're at a steakhouse.

Dine-Out Devils Survival Guide

Wouldn't it be nice to have an angel on your shoulder suggesting exactly what you should choose from any menu? Here are some pointers on how to dine out with your health and weight in mind:

Universal Restaurant Strategies

➤ Know your cuisine triggers. If you know, for example, that Mexican is a trigger for you, try to push for the French bistro when you're making plans, especially in the first three weeks of your diet. Try to take an active role in the restaurant selection. If someone suggests Mexican, you can always say, "I had Mexican yesterday."

➤ Have two FiberRich or GG crackers and drink eight ounces of water before you go out to curb your appetite.

➤ Check the menu ahead of time; pick a couple of smart options in case the menu has changed.

➤ Before you arrive, choose your Angel Carb. This may be in the dish itself, such as a sauce, grains or potatoes, an extra glass of wine or a shared dessert (this last is also best to do after the first three weeks in the plan).

➤ Bread *is* the Devil: Skip the breadbasket!

➤ Make only one special request of the chef (if any).

➤ Take a sip of your drink for a toast and save the rest to enjoy during the appetizer or entrée.

➤ Slow down. Put your fork and knife down at least three times, have your water glass filled up three times, and be the talker.

➤ Choose grilled, roasted or baked foods.

➤ The perfect finish to your meal is peppermint tea. It gives you a nice minty taste which helps put a stop to picking and tasting any other desserts on the table, and it gives you something to do with your hands.

➤ Your kitchen is closed! The food and wine and relaxing experience of dining out can soften your resolve and tempt you into saving your dessert for home. You can imagine why this is a very bad idea. When you get home after a dinner out, there's no kitchen reentry except perhaps for a mug of tea.

Best Restaurant Orders by Cuisine

Here is a handy guide to making the best choices from a host of popular restaurant cuisines, from American to Thai. I've suggested the best "type" of order—Stealth, Hungry and Lean—to help you choose no matter what your hunger level or social situation.

STEALTH ORDER. This is a diet-friendly choice for those times— business entertaining, meeting new people—when you don't want to call attention to yourself and make a fuss about eating clean.

No Weigh!

If you wake up feeling hugely fat after a big dinner out, don't torture yourself by jumping on the scale. It's just going to depress you and prompt a bad eating day. If you feel bloated, check out my Recovery Strategies like a Protein Day or Volume-Controlled Day (page 73). Don't let one dinner unravel your progress.

HUNGRY ORDER. This is a good choice for the volume eater— the person who likes or needs a lot of food to feel full, is a fast eater or may just simply be having a hungry day. This is a good choice for those who have twenty pounds or more to lose.

LEAN ORDER. This is the lowest calorie, cleanest choice and it's good for those who want to power through on their goals, are on the final stretch and have just a couple more pounds to go or are struggling with a plateau. It's also good for a night when you are with your best friend or your spouse and you want to eat really clean. This is a good choice for those with only five to ten pounds to lose.

American

➤ **APPETIZER:** Any starter salad with vinaigrette-based dressing. Men have the optional protein appetizers to choose from such as a shrimp cocktail, the raw bar, grilled calamari or tuna tartare.

➤ **ENTRÉE:** A whole roasted fish or other grilled or roasted lean protein (veal, lamb or poultry). If you must have that piece of red meat, be sure to start with just a salad. Remember that when the dish is cooked in marinara, sweet, thickened or brown sauces you have to count this as your carb.

➤ **SIDES:** Any sautéed or steamed vegetable, without sauce.

STEALTH ORDER: Tuna tartare or any dressed salad is fine; scallops are also a good choice—they don't give you very many, they usually come over risotto, but if you have the discipline to just eat the scallops and the few veggies no one notices the carb that's left on your plate.

HUNGRY ORDER: Salad to start and whole grilled fish—takes forever to fillet yourself; order two side vegetables (make at least one of them steamed).

LEAN ORDER: Raw bar or shrimp cocktail or tuna carpaccio and a simple mixed green salad.

Breakfast or Brunch

➤ Egg white omelet with one slice of cheese and two vegetables and a salad. Replace the home fries with an optional side of fruit salad or two slices Canadian bacon.

➤ Oatmeal made with water and small fruit salad.

➤ two poached eggs with lettuce and tomato, one slice dry toast and fruit salad.

➤ Eggs Benedict: no hollandaise sauce and the English muffin will be your carb.

➤ Eggs Florentine (nice because it has the additional spinach): no potato and no hollandaise sauce.

STEALTH ORDER: Eggs Benedict or eggs Florentine, sauce on the side or no sauce, ½ English muffin; skip potatoes (order sauce on the side, even though you will not eat it).

HUNGRY ORDER: Egg white omelet with veggies (goat or mozzarella or one slice American is OK); ask for salad instead of home fries and share side of Canadian bacon or sometimes at brunch you'll see lunch or salad options and there may be a clean protein or veg salad that looks like it will take longer to eat and be more filling.

LEAN ORDER: two poached eggs with sliced tomatoes and berries on the side.   ·

BBQ

➤ **APPETIZER:** Mixed green salad, peel 'n' eat shrimp (may be salty).

➤ **ENTRÉE:** Blackened catfish, smoked or rotisserie chicken (go for ¼ of a chicken; no skin); with ribs always go dry rubbed and ask for the leanest cut (Memphis style is best).

➤ **SAUCE TIP:** Best sauce is the one that is more vinegar/spice and less tomato/sugar.

➤ **SIDES:** Collard greens, coleslaw (if it is vinegar based!), green beans, baked beans (count as carb—best side when chicken or shrimp or fish are protein choices for meal).

➤ **DEVILS:** Cornbread, hushpuppies (fried cornbread), fatty sugary ribs (St. Louis spare ribs are fattiest), fried catfish, beef brisket, pulled pork.

STEALTH ORDER: Peel 'n' eat shrimp or any salad and for entrée go for dry-rubbed ribs (leanest cut), sides of collard greens and coleslaw.

HUNGRY ORDER: Any salad and then go for ¼–½ chicken (depending on appetite), no skin and pick three side veggies—see above.

LEAN ORDER: Mixed greens (ask for dressing on the side, no cheese) and entrée is either peel 'n' eat shrimp or blackened catfish with just steamed collard greens.

Chinese

➤ **APPETIZER:** Small (or cup) hot-and-sour or egg-drop soup (for those who are not salt sensitive).

➤ **ENTRÉE:** Any dish with a steamed protein and veggies. You can also pick the vegetable of your choice (if you get tired of the broccoli, switch it out with bok choy). Ask for the sauce on the side, no sugar, cornstarch, or MSG.

➤ **ENTRÉE:** Steamed moo shoo chicken. Add ½ of the container of Hoisin sauce and add light (low-sodium) soy sauce.

➤ **ENTRÉE:** For those with thirty plus to drop, if you can, share ½ Peking duck, skip the pancake and sauce and get a side steamed veggie of your choice.

➤ **SIDES:** Pick either brown rice or a fist-sized portion of either steamed vegetable or shrimp dumplings to count as your carb.

➤ **DEVILS:** Avoid sweet-and-sour protein choices: They're often deep-fried. Avoid egg rolls and crunchy noodles and skip the sesame/General Tsao's/lo mein options.

➤ **NOTES:**

- Eat all meals with chopsticks to help slow you down.

- When eating Chinese out at a restaurant, try to request one steamed dish if you can, but if you can't, the key is to skip the rice/noodle dishes because the sauces will count as your carb. Also make sure with each course you fill your plate with 50%–75% veggies and the rest protein—and no seconds.

Be sure to drink an extra liter of water after dinner to help with the sodium.

- See box family-style rules, page 223.

STEALTH ORDER: Hot-and-sour soup (salty, low cal), shared ½ Peking duck (skip the sauce and pancake) and veggies added from other dishes at the table. Chicken or shrimp and broccoli also work and the sauce is your carb; skip the rice.

HUNGRY ORDER: Soup plus 1–2 spare ribs plus any chicken/shrimp/veg dish steamed or moo shoo steamed. Also look for whole fishes that are simply prepared; you can always request sauce on the side.

LEAN ORDER: Look for the "diet" section; most Chinese restaurants now have a special steamed section, making this very easy. Get the wonton soup but just eat the broth (skipping the starter altogether is the best option) and go for steamed chicken/shrimp and broccoli or bok choy or the moo shoo steamed, no pancake. (These are good choices when ordering in; you can always use your own mustard or hot sauce to spice it up.)

French Bistro

➤ **APPETIZER:** Arugula and shaved parmesan salad, mixed green salad with goat cheese, oysters on the half shell, shrimp cocktail, French onion soup (hold the bread and cheese; not for salt sensitive).

➤ **ENTRÉES:** Grilled fish and veggies, steak with salad (no frites), moules in white wine/garlic broth (no frites; ask for salad instead).

Two appetizers in place of one entrée: a salad and either oysters, shrimp cocktail, moules, and tuna tartar.

But be sure to add 1–2 sides of steamed or sautéed vegetables to help fill you up.

➤ **SIDES:** Steamed or sautéed vegetables.

➤ **DEVILS:** Watch out for the beurre blanc sauce added to a lot of fish entrées; ask for it on the side.

STEALTH ORDER: Start with French onion soup (pick around the crouton and cheese) and the roasted chicken, which usually comes with julienne veggies and roasted potatoes; take off the skin on the chicken and pick around the potatoes.

HUNGRY ORDER: Start with fruit de mer (raw bar tower; skip the butter or mayo on the side) or mixed green salad and go for steamed mussels in white wine/garlic; ask for veggies instead of frites.

LEAN ORDER: Share some raw bar and do the tuna Nicoise salad for the entrée.

Greek or Mediterranean

➤ **APPETIZER:** Tomato and cucumber salad or Greek salad (without the grape leaves; best for those with more than thirty to lose).

➤ **ENTRÉE:** Choose grilled fish or grilled chicken or shrimp kabob.

➤ **SIDES:** Choose one carb. Hummus with ¼ pita or 1 fist of rice with entrée if you can handle yourself. I only recommend this for those who have good self-discipline. (Hummus can be the devil for some so be cautious with this one.)

STEALTH ORDER: Tomato and cucumber salad (also share in the pita and hummus; see rule above) plus chicken or shrimp kabob (skip the rice that might come with your entrée).

HUNGRY ORDER: Grilled octopus or Greek salad (fat in cheese will be more filling). Whole grilled fish is a good choice; add a side of green vegetables if possible.

LEAN ORDER: Tomato and cucumber salad and grilled octopus appetizer for the entrée.

Indian

➤ **APPETIZER:** Rasam soup or mixed green salad.

➤ **ENTRÉE:** Chicken tikka (not tikka masala) or chicken or shrimp tandoori.

➤ **SIDE:** ½ roti bread, 1 fist rice or 2 pappadum will be your carb.

➤ **DEVILS:** Tikka masala, samosas, vegetable pakora, naan bread.

STEALTH ORDER: ½ roti or 2 pappadum plus ½ fist of dahl (this is a 2-carb meal) and chicken tikka (skip the rice).

HUNGRY ORDER: Mixed green salad or rasam soup plus chicken or shrimp tikka (can get extra raita—yogurt—sauce) and share a side of palak paneer (this spinach dish may have more or less fat depending on how it's prepared).

LEAN ORDER: Rasam soup and tandoori vegetable.

Italian

➤ **APPETIZER:** Any version of a salad with shaved parm or pecorino. Minestrone soup if not salt sensitive. Look for protein apps like tuna tartare, grilled octopus or prosciutto with melon.

➤ **ENTRÉE:** Shrimp marinara (sauce is the carb), chicken scarpariello (sauce is the carb) or grilled fish (or another protein grilled) of the day plus a side order of any green vegetable (steamed if possible). You can also always have a veal or chicken Milanese (and ask for it without breading). Steak tagliata—grilled skirt steak, lean cut—is good for those with thirty plus to lose.

➤ **DEVIL:** Cream sauces, anything "alfredo," pasta dishes. Watch the eggplant parm—this veggie is known for soaking up the oil!

➤ See special on family-style rules below.

STEALTH ORDER: Starter salad and shrimp marinara, chicken scarpariello or steak tagliata (just skip the potatoes)—if any entrée comes with pasta don't have them remove it, just skip it.

HUNGRY ORDER: Start with salad (or grilled octopus or tuna tartare) or even insalata caprese (thirty plus to lose) and have the veal or chicken Milanese without the breading plus side green veggie.

LEAN ORDER: Two apps—go for arugula salad plus grilled calamari or another lean protein appetizer and side veggie. Alternatively, choose any simple, grilled fish as entrée.

Japanese

➤ **APPETIZER:** Miso soup (for those who are not salt sensitive) or mixed green salad with half serving of the ginger dressing.

➤ **ENTREE:** Chicken or salmon teriyaki with double steamed veggies (no rice, sauce is your carb) or six-piece maki roll (Angel Carb) with four pieces sashimi or six pieces of sashimi and side order oshitashi (spinach).

➤ Look for rolls wrapped in cucumber instead of rice (naruto style).

➤ Edamame usually comes salted and it is soy beans, so this works best for vegetarians or slower eaters who will only have a few pieces.

➤ You can also always sub the rice in a hand roll with cucumber.

➤ **DEVILS:**

Tempura, spider, dynamite, spicy rolls, and eel; dishes described as Agemono or tempura, both of which are deep fried; sushi rolls made with cream cheese and too much avocado.

➤ Always request lite soy sauce and add wasabi and ice cubes to help dilute it and no refills! (If you're salt sensitive use lemon only.)

➤ Eat with chopsticks to help slow you down.

➤ Be careful with sake: It is more calories than you think! Six ounces of sake is about 240 calories versus 150 calories for six ounces of wine.

Calorie Roll Call	Calories
Cucumber roll	110
Avocado roll	140
Tuna roll	185
California roll (only do this when you aren't having additional sashimi)	255
Spicy tuna (skip this)	290
Eel avodaco (skip this)	372

STEALTH ORDER: Miso soup, one tuna cucumber roll and four pieces sashimi; side of oshitashi.

HUNGRY ORDER: Share edamame, salad (just use ½ ginger dressing), one yellowtail with scallion hand roll, four pieces of sashimi, side of oshitashi and add on miso at the end (that's the way it is done in Japan and it's nice to end with warm filling soup for those who aren't salt sensitive).

LEAN ORDER: Miso soup (if not salt sensitive). Or choose salad, just use ½ of dressing on side. Six pieces of sashimi, side of oshitashi (skip soy sauce and use lemon on sashimi).

Mexican

➤ **ENTRÉE:** Grilled chicken or shrimp fajita with sautéed vegetables (skip tortilla).

➤ **ENTRÉE:** Soft taco on corn tortilla—2 soft tacos = one carb. Go with chicken or shrimp and add salsa, a little avocado and some beans (skip the sour cream and cheese).

  • Always ask for sliced jicama instead of chips.

➤ **DEVILS:** Sour cream and cheese. (Go easy on the guacamole: avocado is a healthy fat but the calories add up fast);

  • The margarita—choose a light beer instead.

  • Taco salad—loaded with cheese, sour cream, the fried shell, this is a calorie bomb!

➤ **NOTES:**

  • Choose your one carb before you arrive (for chips with salsa, place handful of chips on side plate and no additional chips, eat only a fist-sized portion of rice or beans).

STEALTH ORDER: Handful of chips (that's the carb) plus gua-camole, chicken or shrimp fajita and skip the tortilla, rice, beans and eat all your veggies. Or, no chips to start and then do two soft corn tacos (chicken or shrimp), skip the cheese/sour cream/beans and rice when you make them.

HUNGRY ORDER: Ask for jicama to start instead of chips if there is guacamole on the table and go with a clean green salad for an appetizer. Have the chicken or steak fajita if you are re-ally hungry—the fat in the protein will help fill you up faster. Also go for the light beer as your alcohol choice, since you'll feel full from the bubbles.

LEAN ORDER (HIGH-END MEXICAN): start with salad and do ceviche entrée.

Pizza

- ➤ **ENTREE:** Two slices thin crust pizza with vegetables (counts as two carbs) and a side salad (without cheese).

- ➤ **DEVILS:** Extra toppings such as pepperoni, meats and extra cheese; avoid the eggplant parmesan and chicken parmesan sometimes offered at pizza joints—too much fat, salt, carbs, calories.

STEALTH ORDER: One thin-crust slice for women, two for men, plus any salad ordered for table.

HUNGRY ORDER: Same as stealth plus a side of cooked veggies (broccoli, mushrooms).

LEAN ORDER: Skip the pizza altogether and get an entrée salad (many pizza joints have grilled chicken, and you can add it to the salad).

Sports Bar or Bar

➤ **APPETIZER:** Get a light beer, if everyone gets wings, pick at the celery and carrots and have at the most one wing (that will cost you 100 calories, and that's without the blue cheese!).

➤ **ENTRÉES:** Grilled chicken Caesar salad (balsamic vinaigrette), a topless burger or burger without bun (skip the cheese, mayo, bacon), veggie chili, grilled chicken sandwich.

➤ **SIDES:** Any side of green veggies as well as a simple baked potato are always good choices.

Bar Banned	Calories
Cheese fries with creamy/cheesy dressing	2070
Chicken quesadilla	1830
Classic nachos with pico de gallo and sour cream	1450
Buffalo wings with blue cheese dressing (10 wings)	1340
Mozzarella sticks with marinara sauce (9 sticks)	1210

STEALTH ORDER: Burger, plain, take the top off and load up the tomatoes and lettuce on top.

HUNGRY ORDER: Burger no bun and house salad with vinaigrette plus side of green veggies.

LEAN ORDER: Grilled chicken salad (with oil and vinegar) or veggie soup and salad or do a veggie night at a bar (baked potato with some mustard or salsa and add two sides of steamed veggies).

Steakhouse

➤ **APPETIZER:** Any starter salad or the raw bar.

➤ **ENTRÉE:** Grilled lean protein. The smallest sized filet mignon (8–10 oz) is the best lean choice. Alternatively, look for grilled fish; steakhouses usually have excellent simply prepared fish.

➤ When grass-fed beef is on the menu, go for it—the meat is leaner and loaded with omega 3s.

➤ **SIDES:** Steamed is best but sautéed vegetables work too. (Skip the creamed.)

➤ Sauce for steak is the peppercorn but best to skip this because steak has more fat naturally and you don't need the additional sauce.

➤ **DEVILS:** Baked potato (opt for double veggies), iceberg wedge, cream sauces or cheese; the rib eye, prime, porterhouse—all too high in fat.

STEALTH ORDER: Mixed green salad, 10 oz filet, sautéed spinach.

HUNGRY ORDER: Shrimp cocktail, 10 oz filet, sautéed spinach and steamed asparagus.

LEAN ORDER: Mixed green salad and grilled tuna with steamed asparagus (or do two apps: mixed greens and shrimp cocktail or tuna tartare and side of veggies).

Tapas

APPETIZER: Tortilla Española, mussels or shellfish (cooked in white wine broth); stick to proteins.

DEVILS: Breaded items, fried items, cream or cheesy items.

NOTE: Try to put in a request for something green or something protein based; with each wave, put food on your plate (try to put on mostly greens and proteins and feel free to fill with items you'll never want to eat); no double dipping.

STEALTH ORDER: It's way too hard to make special orders on a tapas menu, so everyone orders the stealth way! The key is not to go hungry, leave twenty-five percent of food over on each plate of food and look for protein and veggie choices (don't sweat the fat) for each wave of food. Drink extra water that day to help your body handle the extra salt.

Thai

> **APPETIZER:** Tom yum soup (chicken or shrimp or veg) or som tum (green papaya salad) or Thai salad (usually mixed greens, request chili lime dressing), summer roll (one summer roll is one carb, only order this when doing soup/salad pairing).

> **ENTRÉES:** Three appetizers, such as chicken sate (no peanut sauce), Thai salad tom yum soup. Or pick two appetizers and soup plus Thai beef or shrimp salad.
>   Soup to start, share shrimp or chicken in chili basil sauce; no rice (the sauce counts as carb).

> **DEVILS:** Skip pad thai, pla lard prik (crispy whole snapper makes this unhealthy); tofu that's been fried or even sautéed has extra calories because the tofu can hold onto more oil.

STEALTH ORDER: Tom yum soup and shrimp or chicken in chili basil sauce (just skip the rice; sauce is carb).

HUNGRY ORDER: Tom yum soup and one summer roll and then Thai beef salad—beef is lean but it is flavorful and will fill you up. (Summer roll is carb; the volume of the soup, spring roll and beef salad will take a longer time to eat and keep you full.)

LEAN ORDER: Tom yum soup and the green papaya salad with shrimp on top.

Salad Bar Tips and Recipes

A salad bar can be an oasis of healthy eating or a fat trap. Many offices (as well as local delis and restaurants, of course) have extensive salad bars, and sometimes it's hard to make the right choices. Here are the best steps to building a healthy, delicious salad.

1. **THE DARKER THE BETTER:** Choose darker, more nutritious, greens.

2. **PICK YOUR PROTEIN:** Try grilled chicken, roasted or fresh turkey, dry tuna (packed in water), shrimp, tofu (nonmarinated), grilled steak or ham. Vegetarians can choose plain tofu and unseasoned lentils, edamame or beans. Skip cheese unless you have over thirty pounds to lose or are past the first twenty-one days of the Blueprint when you can choose cheese once or twice a week in a small portion.

3. **DEVILS:** Skip corn, beans, peas, chick peas, roasted peppers, marinated mushrooms, caramelized onions, croutons, fried noodles, tortilla strips, sunflower seeds, dried fruit, candied nuts, potato and pasta salads, tuna and chicken salad made with mayo.

4. **EXCEPTIONS:** If you have thirty pounds or more to lose you can add one small amount of optional fat such as olives, raw sliced almonds, sliced avocado, and shredded mozzarella or feta cheese.

5. **DRESS LIGHT:** Always go for the light or low-fat balsamic dressing, using only one small ladle. Adding extra balsamic or red wine vinegar is always an option. Alternatively, choose another light or low-fat dressing but use only ½ a ladle. Or mix your own dressing: balsamic vinegar, a bit of olive oil and Dijon mustard.

6. **A FIBROUS CRUNCH:** Crumble up two FiberRich or GG crackers for added fiber and that satisfactory crunch.

7. **CHOP, CHOP!** The salads always taste best when you have them chopped or mixed up, so if it's an option, ask for yours to be chopped.

Movie Theater Picks

Movies are great fun and they keep you from mindless munching at home. But, and this is a big but, you have to resist the hot buttered popcorn trap, which will set you back nearly 1,700 calories. Candy, while tempting, is a bad choice. It's obviously high in sugar, and the typical movie concession candy package is huge! And who stops before it's empty? Even choices like Twizzlers, Dots, Starburst and Junior Mints range from about 500 to 850 calories. At the high number, that's two dinners! So plan ahead and bring your own. Use your big purse if the theater frowns on imported treats. Following are some good choices. (If you arrive empty handed, look for a child-sized bag of popcorn with no butter. It will cost you about 300 calories.)

	Calories
17 grapes	60
Polly-O String Cheese	80
2 Mini Babybel Light Cheeses	100
Orville Redenbacher Smart Pop! mini bag	100
Ziploc of fresh strawberries (2 cups)	100
Glenny's Soy Crisps (1.3 oz bag)	140
Luna or any bar under 200 calories	200 or less
Popcorn, Indiana gourmet sea salt (2 serving bag, 6 cups)	260 (2 carbs)

Take Me Out to the Ball Game!

But don't buy me some peanuts and Cracker Jacks! Everybody knows that many food choices at ballparks and sporting events are truly Devilish. How about some fried dough? Or a sausage grinder with the works? But you can satisfy your appetite with a few good picks that are pretty universally available at stadiums, concert venues, and arenas across the country. A surprisingly good choice is the all-American hot dog. Get it without the bun (something for the pigeons) and with a squirt of mustard. It's under 400 calories with the bun and counts as a carb. Other workable choices include garden salads, grilled chicken salads, grilled chicken sandwich or veggie burgers. Stick with water as your beverage of choice and cheer on. And don't forget, you can always pack a turkey sandwich or have a healthy meal at home before the game.

Tips:

➤ Bring or buy bottled water.

➤ Have a balanced meal at home or out before the movie.

➤ Don't start eating the snack you have chosen until the movie starts.

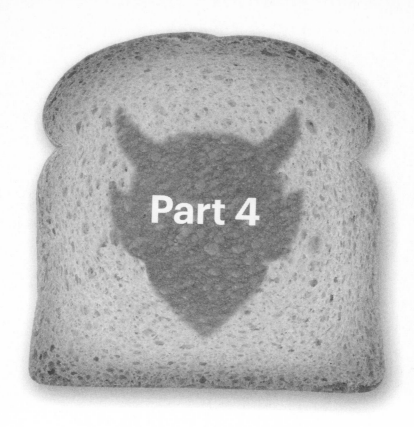

Part 4

Sticking with It

As you go forward with your new healthy eating habits, you may encounter a few speed bumps. Here are a few of the issues that my clients commonly encounter. They have to do with those frustrating plateaus, the issue of maintenance and other common questions.

Plateaus and Tune-Up Techniques

OK, let's say you've been following the Blueprint for a few weeks and you've lost some weight but not as much as you'd like and you don't know what's going on. Or maybe you've been on the Blueprint for a few months and lost a good amount of weight but now you seem to be stuck at a plateau and you're frustrated.

What to do?

First, remember that small changes equal huge success! If you've already made some, you're on your way!

Here are my suggestions that should help you get back on track:

➤ Make it fun / change it up. Working hard to lose weight can get tiresome. You can begin to feel deprived. Or if you reached a plateau you can get to feeling bored and hopeless. Life is a journey and we like to feel we're moving along on an adventure; when we're stuck in one spot we get restless and cranky. Don't let this happen to you! If you are sitting on a fat plateau or if you're feeling discouraged, do something positive to get back on track. Take a new exercise class or hire a personal trainer for a few sessions. Find a diet buddy. Get a new healthy cookbook and experiment each week with one or two new recipes. Can you afford a spa week or weekend? Any of these things can give you a big boost in morale and help you reach your goal.

➤ Get compulsive about your food journal for a week or so. Be brutally honest. Are there picks and sips showing up that are adding up to the culprit calories? Are there nuts and cheese and croutons and bacon bits in your salad? Are you pouring on the dressing?

➤ Control your volume. Focus on your portion sizes. I often find that clients can get too relaxed about the volume of food they're eating. Measure your cereal. Choose yogurt in an individual container. Enjoy oatmeal in packets. Work in some portion-controlled frozen entrées. Don't FreeStyle anything. If you're eating a big salad at lunch, try switching to a Subway sandwich.

➤ Brown-bag it. Sometimes it's hard to control what the deli is serving up even if you think you're making a healthy order. Make your own, like turkey on Arnold's 100-calorie sandwich thins with mustard and lettuce.

➤ Drink more water! This really can help. I've seen it time and again.

➤ Snack carefully. Are you snacking too much? Try cutting out your snacks and see how it goes. If you definitely need a snack, try to reduce the amount and go for the lowest calorie snacks like a 130-calorie bar or a piece of fruit. Watch the timing of your snacks: Be sure you're having them at the most useful strategic time, not just when you're bored or distracted.

➤ Check out your exercise. Are you overexercising? It happens. Clients get a little too compulsive about hitting the gym and their appetite soars. It becomes just too difficult to keep their calorie intake low because they're absolutely *starving!* If this describes you, lighten up on the exercise for a time. Reduce the length or intensity of your workout or alternate power workouts with more relaxed exercise days.

➤ Have you become a lazy exerciser? Invest in a heart rate monitor and push yourself a bit. If your exercise doesn't seem to boost your appetite, you can afford to boost your activity level a bit. A heart monitor helps you keep track of how you're doing and it also motivates you.

➤ Watch the oil: Pay attention to the dressings you're using on your salads and any added oil in your foods. It's very high in calories and easy to overuse.

➤ Watch the salt. Salt can make your body retain weight and make it harder to lose. Be cautious of foods that contain salt: olives, sardines, nuts, pickles, roasted peppers, anything from a can, frozen foods (switch to the low-sodium versions), V8, deli meats, all cheeses, sauces (even low-sodium soy sauce), cottage cheese, breads. Many clients say to me, salt is just salt: "I'll just sweat it out," but most don't exercise enough anyway and even if they do, salt makes it harder for their body to let go of fat. Increasing water intake helps, but working on salt really does more to get the scale moving down again.

➤ Are you a cream fiend? Sometimes adding too much cream or even milk to your coffee, especially if you have a few coffees daily, can add too many calories to your daily intake. Try substituting tea with nothing but lemon if you like, for any drinks beyond your early morning one. Try substituting milk if you've been using half 'n' half.

➤ Watch your alcohol. Try to cut down on your wine intake: If you routinely have three glasses, make it one or two. If you feel you need to sip something, try diet tonic water with seltzer and lime.

➤ Know your medications. Birth control pills, antidepressants, and other medications can affect your weight. Check with your doctor to see if any of your medications might affect your weight and, if so, if it's possible to switch to a version that won't.

➤ Sleep. Make sure you're getting enough sleep. There's so much research that demonstrates that when you don't get enough sleep, it's harder to lose weight.

➤ Don't forget about Volume-Controlled Days or Protein Days. They're perfect for recovery but also helpful when you hit a plateau.

Maintenance

Most diets these days have a stage they refer to as "maintenance." This is usually a phase where the dieter has reached his or her goal and now moves to a different level of the diet with different choices and options. I'll be honest: I've never really focused on putting people on any kind of maintenance *plan*. In fact, sometimes when my clients reach their goal weight and I encourage them to permit themselves some small indulgence they resist! Why? My plan is a very balanced, easy-to-understand, easy-to-follow eating plan. Its main principles are quite simple: Eliminate Devil Carbs, reduce Angel Carbs, focus on volume, up your water intake and learn to recognize and manage your Devils. It's not hard to live with these principles. Most people struggle a bit during the first twenty-one days to stay on track, but once they've gotten past the first three weeks they're pretty much on autopilot.

So what happens when you reach your goal weight? I wish I could tell you that a big rubber duck will fall out of the sky and quack some congratulations at you. But that probably isn't going to happen. In fact, I should alert you to one risk you'll face when you reach your goal. Don't crack open the champagne the second the needle on your scale hits bingo: I don't count it as a real official weight until you've maintained it for a week. That's because weight does fluctuate constantly and you need to confirm that you really have landed in your sweet spot. In fact, I recommend that you stick with the Blueprint for a full four weeks after initially reaching your goal weight. Once you do that, you really are at your goal! Your body has reached a new set point, and you will probably be able to stay within a few pounds of your goal weight without much difficulty. When this happens, you'll really know what it means to have a new, healthy-eating lifestyle.

And after that? Well, almost every one of my clients has been able to maintain their new weight by simply adding a few Indulgences and a few Angel Carbs into their menu. You're never going to increase your Devil Carbs. You're never going to be drinking racks of piña coladas. And you're never going to be diving into a breadbasket with wild abandon. You know too much now.

If you need some guidelines on how to proceed once you reach your goal, here's what I suggest: Your basic plan remains the same but you can add in one indulgent dinner a week.

What is an Indulgence? It's one component of a meal—pasta, chocolate soufflé, a slice of pizza—anything you want it to be. But not a Plunge. If you know you want the soufflé, you're still going to skip the bread. Your Indulgence equals your carb for the day.

It's best to enjoy your indulgent meal at dinner (because this way you are not set off as you might be at lunch), it must be with people and it needs to be at a restaurant where you can really enjoy a single portion (as opposed to a home-cooked meal where you could go overboard on volume). I also recommend that you pick one thing to indulge in; for example, I would not go for bread, pasta and dessert all in one night. If you want pasta, then have salad, then pasta and then fruit. If you would like a burger, have salad and a burger with the bun and fruit. If you're in the mood for a real dessert, then have a salad, some simple fish and then choose a dessert.

You also have the option at maintenance to up your Angel Carb intake: If you were only having one a day you can now have the option to have two on three days of the week. If you were having two Angel Carbs, you can bump it up to three on two days a week.

> **BLUEPRINT:** 1 Angel Carb per day
> **MAINTENANCE:** 2 Angel Carbs on weekends
>
> **BLUEPRINT:** 2 Angel Carbs per day
> **MAINTENANCE:** 3 Angel Carbs on weekends

Maintenance Treats

Many clients ask me about having a treat after dinner to satisfy a craving once in a while. My rules on after dinner treats are the following:

1. Only after the first twenty-one days on the Blueprint

2. Only under 80 calories and individually wrapped, single portion

3. Only within twenty minutes of dinner

One of my favorite evening treats is my frozen chocolate ice cream. Here's the recipe (there's another recipe for Frozen Strawberry or Banana Smoothie on page 276):

FROZEN CHOCOLATE ICE CREAM   Add 1 cup of unsweetened vanilla almond milk (Blue Diamond), one tablespoon of unsweetened cocoa, 1 teaspoon vanilla extract, 1–2 packets of Splenda and a bunch of ice to the blender. Blend!

Cold Treats

➤ Frozen Dannon Light 'n' Fit yogurt

➤ Frozen Greek yogurt

➤ Ciao Bella blood orange mini sorbet pops

➤ Ciao Bella blood orange mini sorbet cups

➤ Edy's fruit pops

Chocolate Cravings

➤ Chocolite (chocolate crispy caramel)

➤ Bissinger's 100-calorie chocolate bar

➤ Adora dark chocolate calcium

See page 287 for additional suggestions.

Some Common Questions

How Much Weight Can I Expect to Lose?

Everybody is different. In general, two pounds a week is considered a healthy rate of weight loss, but most people don't lose at that rate consistently. There are fast losers and slow losers. I have not recognized any real overall pattern with my clients, but in the end, everybody gets there. If you have never dieted before or have a lot of weight to lose, you could lose as much as five pounds in the first week and then typically average two pounds a week from then on. If you have less weight to lose or if you're a veteran dieter, it's harder to predict your rate of weight loss. Don't be surprised if you don't show much movement on the scale until the second week. Some clients immediately drop a few pounds just because they're eliminating Devil Carbs and drinking their water. Others have never indulged much in Devil Carbs so their weight loss will be a little slower.

How Much Should I Weigh?

I hate this question! No matter what BMI charts and other guidelines tell you, the truth is that you probably know best how much you should weigh.

The first thing I tell clients is not to get too hung up on the number on their scale. Many people know what they want to weigh and already have a goal in their heads. I think it's wise to think back to the last time you felt comfortable in your skin and your clothes. For you, that might be 150 pounds or 115 pounds. But you have to be realistic. I occasionally have clients who become obsessed with a specific number, even after they reach a weight that is great for them. It's a shame to allow

> **Sticky Decades**
>
> This is the term I use when dieters find their scale stuck just at the bottom of "a decade." Many people find that they get stuck at, for example, 151 pounds. They really struggle to break through to the 140s. Sometimes they're stuck for a week or maybe two. If this happens to you, don't worry; just stick with the Blueprint and the number will change. You may find you suddenly land three or four pounds into the new decade.

yourself to be unhappy if you can't reach a goal that may not be realistic for you in the first place. Most of us in our twenties wished we weighed less; as we get older, we look back at our twenty-year-old bodies and would give anything to have it back! So settle on a number or at least a range that will be healthy and comfortable for you; one you can live with but not be obsessed by. If you really are clueless about what your weight should be, it could be useful to have a conversation about it with your doctor.

How Often Should I Weigh Myself?

While it's important to be accountable and to keep track of progress with regular weigh-ins, everyone reacts to a hop on the scale differently. For that reason, I have two answers to this question, depending on how you handle the number on the scale.

If you find it important to check your number every day, if it motivates you to eat well and stay on track, then weigh yourself at the same time every morning. If you like, you can record the number on your food journal.

If, on the other hand, you know that a low or a high number can prompt a bad eating day, then weigh in weekly. You want to avoid either of these scenarios: "Holy good night! I'm up a pound. Damn it. I'm heading for the fridge," or "Yipee! I'm down two. I'm heading for the fridge!" Remember that your clothes can often tell you a lot: When your pants are loose, you are on the right track.

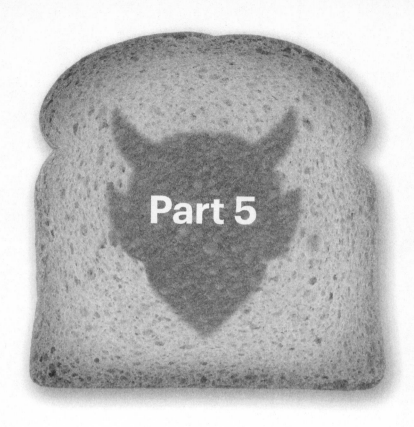

Part 5

Resources

The Ultimate Restaurant Guide

Includes my top pick food choices at fast-food chains,[1] popular restaurant chains[2] and coffee shops.[3]

Applebee's

	Calories
Onion soup	150
Grilled shrimp skewer salad	210
Cajun lime tilapia	310
Steak and portobellos	330
Italian chicken and portobello sandwich	360
Teriyaki steak and shrimp skewers	370
Confetti Chicken	370

Note: All items on special "Weight Watcher's" menu are BID approved. Add on onion soup or side of steamed veggies to any angel meal choice.

Au Bon Pain[4]

	Calories
Ham and Swiss or turkey and Swiss sandwich	320
Egg white cheddar breakfast on wheat skinny bagel	250

1 *Fast-food chains: When you select a sandwich or wrap, count this as one of your Angel Carbs for the day. Also, while I am usually not a fan of wraps and parfaits, you will see that in special situations they work because of the calories per serving.*

2 *When dining at a chain, always check the menu ahead of time to see what looks good to you. Remember who you dine with needs to go into your thought process when you make your meal picks. If it is your best girlfriend who loves to eat clean with you, go with the steamed option, get sauces on the side and be as picky as you want. If it is a first date, you are with a group of people from work or you are with a cut-your-hair friend, it is best to order straight off the menu. No one ever watches how much food you consume, they just watch what you order. Also, in a group situation where you are with trigger friends, for appetizers I recommend against ordering your own special salad to start with while they gorge on wings. Put 2–3 pieces of whatever is ordered on your plate, and eat it very slowly . . . you'll fit in better and no one will notice you.*

3 *For all coffee and tea choices, the best option is hot or cold tea or coffee for 0–5 calories (no additions). If the calories in the drink exceed 60, you must lower the calories in your meal to compensate (or count as a breakfast if over 150 and add fruit). For an afternoon occasional fun snack, you can pick a drink under 200 calories. Note all recommended picks are tall sizes (or ounces where specified); if you choose a larger size, pay attention to the additional calories. Remember that you can save 90+calories by choosing skim milk over whole milk and always choose the sugar-free option.*

4 *Best known for their soups, while they change daily they do have low-sodium, low-fat, vegan and gluten-free options.*

Small oatmeal	170
12-veggie soup, large	240

Burger King

	Calories
Egg and cheese Croissan'wich (without croissant)	150
Side garden salad	40
Side salad with Ken's fat-free ranch dressing	100
Hamburger (without bun)	130
Hamburger (with bun)	260
TenderGrill chicken garden salad (without dressing)	230
TenderGrill chicken garden salad (with Ken's fat-free ranch dressing)	290
Flame-broiled chicken tenders (4 pieces)	145
BK Veggie burger (without mayo)	320

California Pizza Kitchen[5]

	Calories
Tuscan white bean minestrone (cup)	157
Minestrone paired with half roasted vegetable salad	297
Half classic Caesar with chicken or salmon (no croutons and keep Caesar dressing)	500
Full Caesar with grilled chicken or shrimp (with the fat-free vinaigrette)	325
Half roasted vegetable salad with shrimp	393
Wild-caught mahi-mahi with wok-stirred vegetables	586
Kids' grilled chicken with broccoli	246

5 The best picks are the options below, especially during first three weeks of the plan, but if you crave pizza go with the thin-crust roasted artichoke and chicken option and only eat half; count as Angel Carb for day and do it for dinner, skip all appetizers (492 cals). Or if you are with kids, you can order yourself your own kids' traditional cheese (637 cals), leaving over a quarter of the pizza untouched. Everything else on the menu is over 1,000 calories, so stick to the Angel list.

Cheesecake Factory[6]

	Calories
(All Weight-Management Salads):	
Asian chicken salad	570
Spicy chicken salad	510
Pear and endive salad	570

Chili's

	Calories
Side of steamed veggies with parmesan cheese	80
Black bean burger (patty only no bun or topping)	200
Black bean burger (with whole wheat bun)	290
Guiltless salmon (three-quarter rule)	480
Guiltless chicken sandwich (eat half bread)	500

Così[7]

	Calories
Turkey light sandwich (on wheat)	390
Hummus and fresh veggie sandwich (on wheat)	397
Lighter side Così signature salad	378
Bombay chicken salad	168
Shanghai chicken salad	319

Domino's

	Calories
2 thin crust ham/pineapple slices (equals 2 Angel Carbs)	310

6 Bread is the Devil here; it is absolutely delish bread, but if you dine here during first three weeks of the plan, skip it. You'll have it again on maintenance, but for now stick to one of the Angels below. Also, when you order the weight-management salad, you can point to the salad and say, "this Asian chicken salad"—this way it isn't obvious to those with you that you are getting the weight-management option.

7 Be sure to stay away from the bread—don't even sample it! If you order the salad, skip the side bread. If you really crave the bread go for the turkey light or hummus and veggie sandwich on wheat.

Dunkin' Donuts

Hot Drinks	Calories
Tea	0
Coffee (black, 10oz)	15
Any flavored coffee (hazelnut, French vanilla, black)	20
Coffee (with skim milk, 10oz)	25
Vanilla latte lite (10oz)	80

Cold Drinks	Calories
Iced coffee with skim milk (16oz)	25
Iced Latte with skim milk (16oz)	70
Turbo Ice (16oz)	120

Food	Calories
Egg white turkey sausage wake-up wrap	150
Egg white veggie flatbread	280
Egg and cheese on English muffin	320
Ham, egg and cheese wake-up wrap	200
Ham and cheese flatbread	310

Kentucky Fried Chicken (KFC)

	Calories
Roasted chicken Caesar salad (without dressing or croutons)	220
Roasted chicken Caesar salad (with original ranch fat-free dressing)	255
KFC Original Recipe chicken breast (no skin or breading)	160
Tender Roast chicken sandwich (without sauce, skin or breading)	300
Oven Roasted Twister Sandwich (without sauce)	340
Green beans	20

Le Pain Quotidien

Hot Drinks

	Calories
Coffee	8
Pot of tea (green, red fruit, mint)	5
Skim cappuccino	30
Skim latte, large	90

Cold Drinks

	Calories
Iced tea (green and mint)	5
Iced coffee	5
Lemonade iced tea (sweetened w/ raw agave)	40
Mint lemonade (sweetened w/ raw agave)	70

Food

	Calories
1 soft-boiled egg (no bread) and large fruit salad	210
Organic steel-cut oatmeal with berries	210
1 soft-boiled egg with bread	290
Low-fat yogurt and berries	150
Six-vegetable garden gluten-free quiche	370
Smoked salmon with avocado and chopped dill tartine	350
Ricotta with figs tartine	390
Roasted turkey and avocado tartine	400
Tuscan white bean and prosciutto with arugula tartine	420
Quinoa and arugula salad	430
Grilled chicken Cobb salad (without the cheese or bacon and with half the dressing)	400

McDonald's

	Calories
Fruit 'n' Yogurt Parfait	160
Egg McMuffin (without English muffin)	140
Side salad	20
Side Salad (with low-fat balsamic vinaigrette)	60
Fruit and Walnut Salad (snack size)	210
Caesar salad with grilled chicken	220

Caesar salad with grilled chicken	
(with low-fat balsamic vinaigrette)	260
Hamburger	250
Honey Mustard Snack Wrap (with grilled chicken)	260
Asian salad with grilled chicken	300
Asian salad with grilled chicken	
(with low-fat balsamic vinaigrette)	340

Panda Express[8,9]

	Calories
Mixed veggies (8.6 oz)	70
Veggie spring roll (1 piece)	90
Hot-and-sour soup	110
Mushroom chicken (5.9 oz)	220
Broccoli beef	130
Chicken breast with string beans	170

Panera Bread[10]

	Calories
French onion soup (no cheese or croutons; 8 oz)	80
Low-fat chicken noodle soup (8 oz)	100
Low-fat vegetarian black bean soup (8 oz)	110
Classic café salad	170
Half Asian sesame salad (without dressing)	200
Half Asian sesame salad (with reduced-sugar Asian sesame vinaigrette)	245
Half Fuji apple salad with chicken (without dressing)	260
Half Fuji apple salad with chicken (with reduced fat balsamic vinaigrette)	320
Half smoked turkey breast sandwich on Country bread	220
Fresh fruit cup (small)	60

8 When choosing the hot-and-sour soup, add another Angel option such as the mixed veggies or veggie spring roll to make it a full meal.

9 All chicken, beef and shrimp dishes listed are served as 5.5 oz portions unless otherwise indicated. Steamed rice (8 oz) is 380 calories.

10 If you are choosing a soup, add only the classic café house salad to make it a complete meal.

P.F. Chang's[11]

	Calories
Vegetarian lettuce wraps	140
Egg-drop soup	60
Sweet-and-sour chicken	370
Chang's lemon scallops	243
Buddha's feast, steamed	55

Pizza Hut

	Calories
1 slice 14" Thin 'n' Crispy Pizza, Veggie Lover	240
2 slices 12" Fit 'n' Delicious Pizza, green pepper, red onion, diced red tomato	300
2 slices 12" Fit 'n' Delicious Pizza, ham and pineapple	320
2 slices 12" Fit 'n' Delicious Pizza, diced chicken, mushroom and jalapeño	340

Quiznos

	Calories
Small honey bourbon chicken	270
Small honey bourbon chicken (with Zesty Grille Sauce)	315
Half oven-roasted Turkey Toasty (without dressing)	280
Half oven-roasted Turkey Toasty (with cheese)	325
Cantina chicken flatbread sammie	230
Cantina chicken flat bread sammie (with dressing)	275
Veggie Sammy Flatbread Sammie	200
with Cheese and Dressing	340
Raspberry Vinaigrette Chicken Salad (without Bread and Dressing)	120
with Dressing	250
with Bread	330

11 *Reminder: Every dish is family style, so most dishes are meant for three people, on average, but the calories shown here are per serving. My ultimate pick would be to either have a vegetarian meal and start with the lettuce wraps and choose the Buddha's feast and an egg-drop soup for your entrée, or if you are craving meat opt for just the chicken or the scallop dishes.*

Starbucks

Hot Drinks[12]	Calories
Brewed Tazo teas	0
Brewed coffee / caffè americano (black)	5–10
Espresso (solo)	5
Nonfat cappuccino (best to order extra dry)	60
Nonfat caffè misto	60
Cocoa cappuccino (8 oz)	70
Skinny vanilla latte	90
Skinny caramel macchiato	100
Skim latte (grande)	130
Heather's hot beverage recipe: venti tea with 2 Chai tea bags, add some skim and a Splenda	30

COLD DRINKS	Calories
Iced coffee (freshly brewed over ice, no milk)	5
Nonfat iced sugar-free vanilla latte	60
Frappuccino light blended coffee (various flavors)	110–40
Heather's cold beverage recipe: venti, half iced green tea, half lemonade (request no syrup) and add Splenda	60

FOOD	Calories
Starbucks Perfect Oatmeal	140
Starbucks Perfect Oatmeal (with nuts)	240
Egg white, spinach and feta wrap	280
Reduced fat turkey bacon with egg white on English muffin	320
Greek yogurt honey parfait	300
Farmer's market salad	230
Chicken on flatbread with hummus artisan snack plate	250
Roasted vegetable panini	350
Turkey and Swiss sandwich	390
Protein artisan snack plate	370
Variety of Kind bars	180

12 *While it isn't on the menu, you can order any drink in a "short," 8-ounce size to cut back on additional calories; you can also add in a scoop of protein powder for 30 calories and 6 grams to make the drink a little more filling.*

Subway[13,14]

	Calories
Egg Muffin Melt (egg white and cheese)	140
Low-fat salad (ham, roast beef, oven-roasted chicken, club, turkey breast or Veggie Delite)	150
Low-fat salad (with fat-free Italian dressing)	185
6" low-fat sub (includes 9-grain wheat bread), Veggie Delite	230
6" low-fat sub, turkey breast	280
6" low-fat sub, black forest ham	290
6" low-fat sub, turkey breast and black forest ham	300
6" low-fat sub, roast beef	310
6" low-fat sub, oven-roasted chicken	320

Taco Bell[15]

	Calories
Grilled steak soft taco ("Fresco")	150
Ranchero chicken soft taco ("Fresco")	160
Beef soft taco ("Fresco")	180
Gordita Supreme chicken	270

TGI Friday's[16,17]

	Estimated Calories
Dragonfire Chicken (low-fat)	435
Zen Chicken pot stickers (low-fat; the dumpling counts as your Angel Carb for the day)	500
Shrimp Key West (low-carb)	225

13 *Subway now has a line of healthy meals called Subway Fresh Fit Meals, which include a side of fruit (35 calories for apple slice packet) and a bottle of water. Calorie info below is for salads and sandwiches only.*

14 *These do not include dressing or sauces. Try mustard or vinegars to keep calories low.*

15 *Menu includes "fresco style" items, which contain 10 grams of fat or less.*

16 *TGI Friday's doesn't list their nutrition information for their dishes, that's why you will not see a devils section for TGI Friday's. However, they do have low-fat and low-carb options on the menu. There are salad options not listed on their low-fat or low-carb section that are a good choice that need just a few modifications. Follow the ¾ rule to cut additional calories.*

17 *Also, Friday's features six new entrées for the new Right Portion, Right Price ($6.99–$8.99) menu. However, only two of the offerings, Dragonfire Chicken and Shrimp Key West are BID-approved.*

Sizzling chicken and vegetables (low-carb) (meant for 2 people)	535
Strawberry Fields salad with chicken (no pecans and dressing on the side)	400
Caesar salad with cedar-seared salmon (no croutons and balsamic vinaigrette on the side)	350
Bistro sirloin salad (no corn, balsamic vinaigrette on the side)	450
House salad	210

Wendy's

	Calories
Apple pecan chicken salad (without dressing or pecans)	180
Apple pecan chicken salad (with fat-free French dressing)	220
Chili, small	220
Wendy's Jr. hamburger	230
Grilled chicken Go Wrap	260

Recipes

Here are some very quick and very easy recipes that are Blue-print friendly. All are for a single serving unless otherwise specified, but of course they can easily be multiplied.

Angel Blintzes

I've made these for both breakfast and dinner. Whip together 4 to 6 egg whites until a lot of air is incorporated into the eggs (about 4 minutes). Add a dash of cinnamon and a splash of vanilla extract. You can add some Splenda, too, if you like. Pour into a nonstick omelet pan and, when eggs firm up, spread 2 tablespoons of skim ricotta or whipped cottage cheese and 2 tablespoons of blueberries onto the eggs. Flip or roll up and continue cooking for a minute or so until the eggs have completely cooked through. Enjoy with another sprinkling of cinnamon and 2 FiberRich crackers.

Oatmeal Pancakes

Take a packet of plain instant oatmeal and mix with 4 egg whites, a sprinkle of cinnamon, 2 tablespoons of whipped cottage cheese. Pour into a skillet to create whatever size pancake pleases you and cook until bubbles form on top. Turn and cook until done.

Best Burrito

Mix about 1 cup of Egg Beaters with about ¼ cup of salsa or Desert Pepper black bean dip, plus 2 tablespoons of shredded, low-fat cheese. Roll up in a *BID*-approved tortilla.

Fish in a Package

Take a nonfishy fish fillet like sole or tilapia or orange roughy. Put it on top of a piece of parchment paper (or aluminum foil) that is large enough to fully wrap the fish. Top with chopped cherry tomatoes, 1 tablespoon of capers, and a sprinkle of freshly ground pepper. Close up the parchment or foil, place the package on a baking sheet, and bake in a 375-degree oven for about 20 minutes. Serve on top of steamed spinach. It can also be served with a baked sweet potato.

Wild Salmon in the Toaster Oven

Take a 4 oz piece of wild salmon and take a pinch of salt and pepper and squeeze of lemon and place on top of aluminum foil (that has been sprayed with Pam) on the baking sheet in the toaster oven. Broil the salmon for about 7 minutes until it is cooked through (but pink inside). You can also try with some Dijon mustard on top as an alternative. Serve with steamed veggies and a baked sweet potato.

Super Scallops (Serves 2)

Use 6 large sea scallops. Wrap each scallop around its
perimeter with a thin slice of prosciutto. Sprinkle with
pepper. Heat a skim of olive oil in a nonstick pan and
add a crushed garlic clove. Sauté the scallops in the
hot pan for 2 to 3 minutes on each side, just until firm.
Serve with brown rice and a green vegetable. This is
delicious!

Broiled Fish Raita

Broil any fish. Serve with a sauce of drained Greek yogurt
(reduced fat) with chopped cucumber, minced onion and
cayenne.

Eggplant Parmesan

Slice eggplant pieces into 1-inch circles. Brush with olive
oil and sprinkle with salt. Bake in 350-degree oven for
about 10 minutes. Then add marinara sauce and part-skim
mozzarella and Parmesan cheese. Bake for an additional
20 minutes, or until eggplant becomes soft.

Nicoise Salad

Lightly steam haricots verts, green beans or asparagus.
Arrange on a plate with chickpeas, good canned tuna,
hard-boiled eggs, lettuce, sliced cucumber and tomato.
Dress with oil and vinegar.

Gourmet Tuna Salad

Good canned tuna (packed in olive oil), capers, dill or parsley, lemon juice. Add in rinsed cannellini beans.

Tuna Melt

Preheat broiler. Combine drained chunk light tuna, 1 shallot, 2 tablespoons of low-fat mayonnaise, lemon juice, parsley, salt, a dash of hot sauce and pepper in a medium bowl. Spread ¼ cup of the tuna mixture on each slice of toast (use *BID*-approved bread listed on p 279); top with tomato slices and 2 tablespoons of sharp cheddar cheese. Place sandwiches on a baking sheet and broil until the cheese is bubbling and golden brown, 3 to 5 minutes.

Sizzling Fajitas (Serves 2)

Heat 1 tablespoon olive oil in a medium skillet. Add ½ red or white onion (sliced), 1 sliced pepper, and 2 cloves minced garlic and sauté briefly. Add 8 ounces lean ground beef or turkey meat, reduce heat to medium, and sauté until no longer pink, about 10 minutes. Stir in salsa and chili powder to taste. Sauté for 5 or more minutes. Spread 1 tablespoon reduced-fat plain Greek yogurt in a thin layer on each tortilla. Divide the meat mixture on top of 4 whole wheat tortillas, sprinkle each with part-skim mozzarella cheese, wrap and serve.

Angel Chicken Paillard

Buy thin sliced boneless chicken breast or lightly pound the chicken so it is flat. Then dip the chicken in egg or Egg Beaters, and then mix real bread or panko breadcrumbs and a little unprocessed bran. Place the breaded chicken in a Pyrex dish and bake for 20 minutes at 425. While the chicken is baking, slice the cherry tomatoes. Take the portabella mushrooms and use olive oil spray to lightly coat them before grilling. Once the mushrooms are done, add balsamic vinegar. When the chicken is done, place it on a plate, adding arugula, cherry tomatoes, and a little bit of chopped garlic and balsamic vinegar on top. The mushrooms are an excellent side dish.

Chicken Parm Light

Dip a boneless, skinless chicken breast in flavored Egg Beaters, then dip it in a bowl of unprocessed bran (or Fiber One or All-Bran cereal that's been whirled in the processor or blender) to coat. (Or skip this step and use a Bell & Evans low-fat, breaded chicken breast). Bake in a Pyrex or other type of dish in a preheated 425-degree oven until the chicken is cooked through. In the last 10 minutes of cooking, cover with one-half cup marinara sauce and sprinkle with shredded, low-fat cheese. Serve over steamed spinach or shirataki noodles.

Mustard-Crusted Steak

Marinate a filet mignon or a lean flank or sirloin steak in the following marinade: minced garlic, a tablespoon of Dijon mustard, a tablespoon of Worcestershire sauce, and freshly ground pepper. Leave steak in the marinade for a half hour or so. Broil the steak until done to your liking. Serve with a green veggie. Any leftover flank or sirloin steak can be thinly sliced and served on greens for a delicious lunch salad.

Maintenance Dessert Recipes

To be enjoyed after the initial twenty-one day Blueprint.

➤ *Frozen Chocolate Ice Cream:* 1 cup of unsweetened vanilla almond milk (Blue Diamond), one tablespoon of unsweetened cocoa, 1 teaspoon vanilla extract, 1–2 packets of Splenda and a bunch of ice; combine all in blender.

➤ *Frozen Strawberry or Banana Smoothie:* 1 cup unsweetened vanilla almond milk (Blue Diamond), 5 frozen strawberries or ½ banana and a bunch of ice; combine all in blender.

Fast Cooking Tips

How Do I Hard-Boil an Egg?

Put the eggs in water, put the heat on high. Once the water is boiling, set the timer for 10 minutes. Turn off the heat after the timer goes off. Pour out the hot water and pour cold water over the eggs. Let them cool, peel now to enjoy or save them in their shell to eat later or on another day!

How Do I Bake a Sweet or White Potato?

Poke it a few times with a fork, cook it for 11 minutes in the microwave and you are done!

What's a Super Easy Way to Cook Fish?

The fastest way is to line a baking sheet with aluminum foil. Spray some Pam on the foil, then put the fish on top, with a little pepper and lemon and a tiny dash of salt. Broil for 7–8 minutes in the toaster oven.

How Do I Steam Veggies Really Quickly?

Clean the veggies, put them in a glass container, wet a paper towel and place it on top of the veggies, then place the lid on top. Place the container in the microwave and cook on high for 4–6 minutes depending on the vegetable and your microwave—this works for everything from broccoli to asparagus to sliced portobello mushrooms.

Shopping List

Food shopping is an important component of weight loss. Making the right choices in the supermarket means that you'll have delicious, healthy, satisfying food to put on the table. I've always felt that a big part of my job as a nutritionist is being able to steer people to the best choices available, whether they're looking for a condiment or a healthy frozen meal. My shopping list is a compilation of my best recommendations. They are all taste-tested and approved by my family, my clients and me.

You'll notice that the shopping list is arranged by my food categories. This is so it will be simple for you to find anything you're looking for when you follow my diet. So all the snacks, frozen dinners, fibers and so on are grouped together.

One warning on warehouse-type shopping: While we all love the big box food stores, beware of loading up on too much food or on unhealthy food. It's easy to convince yourself that a car-sized box of granola is a great idea. But if it's going to sit in your cabinet for you to munch on mindlessly for the next six months until you're so sick of it (and you're wearing three-quarters of it on your butt) that you throw it out, it's not really a bargain, is it? My husband and I have learned this lesson the hard way. We now try to restrain ourselves at the big box: toilet paper, yes; five pounds of pistachios, no. And, of course, you know never to go food shopping hungry. And never, ever take a sample!

Shopping List

Angel Carbs

Breads
✓ Whole wheat, sprouted grains, flax
✓ Ingredients to look for: whole wheat flour, unbleached
✓ Ingredients to avoid: HFCS, molasses, sugars, dyes, preservatives, enriched white flour
✓ Brands: Damascus Bakeries Flax Roll-ups, Thomas' Light Multi-Grain English Muffins, Arnold's Select Sandwich Thins (100 calories), La Tortilla Factory high-fiber wheat wrap, Nature's Own 100% whole wheat bread (sugar-free)

Whole Grains
✓ Whole grains are easy to store and have a long shelf life, so there is no reason not to buy them in bulk to cut down on costs.
✓ Remember when cooked the serving size on all is ½ cup cooked
✓ Grains: amaranth, bulgur wheat, kamu, millet, quinoa, farro
✓ Brands: Bob's Red Mill, DeBoles, Kretschmer wheat germ

Breakfast Choices
✓ Waffles
• Brands: Van's Natural Foods Waffles Lite (gluten-free version available), Kashi Go Lean Original Seven-Grain Waffles
✓ Muffins
• Brands: VitaMuffin MultiBran 100-calorie muffin

Pasta Substitutes (Count as Veggie, Not Carb)
✓ Brands: kombu seaweed noodles, tofu shirataki noodles (in all varieties)

Pastas (Only Recommended for Maintenance)
✓ Ingredients to look for: whole wheat
✓ Ingredients to avoid: bleached, enriched, white flour
✓ Brands: Deboles whole wheat, Deboles gluten-free multigrain spaghetti, Eden 100% buckwheat noodles, Al Dente All-Natural Carba-Nada egg fettuccine noodles

Fibers

Crackers

✓ Brands: FiberRich Bran Crackers, GG Scandinavian Bran Crispbread (available in convenient 2-cracker packs), Health Valley Original Rice Bran Crackers (GF, W).

NOTE: For those on maintenance or for those who do not like the FiberRich, GG or Health Valley options, the next best choice is Wasa Fiber Rye and Marys Gone Crackers (GF).

Cereals (Breakfast Only; Count as Fiber)

✓ Oatmeals
- Steel-cut (instant or regular)
- Ingredients to look for: whole grain oats
- Ingredients to avoid: caramel color, sugars, preservatives, artificial flavors
- Brands: McCann's instant Irish oatmeal, regular flavor (100-calorie packs); Arrowhead Mills instant oatmeal, plain; Trader Joe's steel-cut oatmeal, instant; Kashi Go Lean creamy oatmeal

✓ Dry Cereal
- Ingredients to look for: wheat brand, oat fiber, whole grain wheat, evaporated cane juice
- Ingredients to avoid: high fructose corn syrup, hydrogenated oils, food coloring, preservatives
- Brands: Kashi Go Lean (*not Crunch!), Uncle Sam's, Nature's Path Organic SmartBran, Mesa Sunrise (GF)

Protein

Eggs

✓ Brands: Country Hen Organic Omega-3's, Organic Valley large brown eggs, Eggology 100% egg whites, Ready Gourmet Easy Omelets (egg white options)

Milk

✓ Ingredients to look for: low-fat, vitamin A, vitamin D, organic
✓ Ingredients to avoid: flavoring, sugar, SPI, artificial flavors, additives, hexane
✓ Brands: Organic Valley, Hemp Dream hemp milk, Silk, Skim Plus, Lactaid, almond milk

Yogurt

✓ Ingredients to look for: live active cultures, grade A pasteurized skimmed milk

✓ Ingredients to avoid: sugars, sweeteners, syrups, high fructose corn syrup, gelatin, flavor

✓ Brands: Fage Total 0% or 2% Greek yogurt, plain or fruit flavored; Stonyfield fat-free yogurt; Silk plain yogurt; Siggi's yogurt, plain or fruit flavored; Siggi's probiotic drink; Chobani 0% or 2% Greek yogurt, plain or fruit flavored

Cheese

✓ Ingredients to look for: cultured pasteurized grade A skim milk

✓ Ingredients to avoid: excess salt, coloring, potato starch, cellulose powder, calcium sulfate, whey, preservatives, annatto and apocarotenal (color), whey protein

- Cottage cheese: Friendship low-fat or fat-free, whipped; Breakstone's 2% individual packs; Breakstone's 100-calorie cottage cheese with fruit on the side
- Cheddar: Cabot mini 50% reduced fat (lactose free) ¾ oz
- Laughing Cow 35-calorie wedge
- Mini Babybel Light cheese rounds
- Horizon organic sliced (low-cal) cheese
- Wholesome Valley Organic mozzarella sliced cheese
- 365 string cheese
- Organic Valley Stringles, low moisture, part skim mozzarella cheese
- Organic Valley reduced-fat shredded cheese

Nuts, Nut Butters, Seeds

✓ Nuts can be extremely expensive, another item you can buy in bulk and freeze because they can stay for months in the freezer. Only buy nuts and nut butter if you know you can eat 10–12 nuts at one time or 1½ T, otherwise buy the individual portioned packs.

✓ Always buy unsalted, raw

✓ Nuts: almonds, Brazil nuts, cashews, hazelnuts, macadamia nuts, peanuts, pecans, pine nuts, pistachios, walnuts

✓ Nut butters:

- Ingredients to look for: organic dry roasted nuts, palm fruit oil

- Ingredients to avoid: molasses, hydrogenated vegetable oil, glycerides, sugar
- Brands: Justin's nut butters (80-calorie individual packets and 200-calorie packs), MaraNatha (GF), Barney Butter (100-calorie packs), 365 (Whole Foods) products, Blue Diamond 100-nut bags, Emerald 100-calorie nut bags

Meat/Poultry/Seafood
✓ Fresh (buy organic when you can)
- Meat:
  - » Beef: sirloin, tenderloin, flank steak, ground beef (95% lean)
  - » Ham: extra-lean ham, pork center loin chops, pork cutlets, ground pork, tenderloin
  - » lamb: lamb loin, lamb chops
- Poultry:
  - » Chicken: skinless chicken breast, cornish hen
  - » Turkey: extra-lean ground turkey, turkey breasts
- Seafood:
  - » Whole fish or fillets: cod, flounder, halibut, mackerel, mahi mahi, red snapper, salmon (wild), sardines, sea bass, sole, tilapia, tuna
  - » Shellfish: clams, king crab, lobster, mussels, scallops, shrimp

✓ Frozen
- Poultry: Chicken or turkey meatballs, grilled chicken breasts (organic)
  - » Brands: Applegate Farms, Bell & Evans, Free Bird
- Seafood: halibut, shrimp, salmon fillets
  - » Brands: Whole Catch, EcoFish, St. Dalfour

✓ Packaged (buy low sodium or organic when available)
- Meat: Applegate Farms ham (slow cooked) deli slices, roast beef deli slices
- Poultry (recommended to buy ¼ lb bags and keep in fridge for easy use): turkey breast (oven-roasted) deli slices, turkey bacon, chicken or turkey hot dogs, turkey jerky
  - » Brands: Applegate Farms, Han's All Natural, SnackMasters, FreeBird Seasoned Grilled Chicken Breast Strips

- Seafood: tuna (albacore, canned chunk light in water), sardines, tuna jerky, salmon jerky
  - » Brands: King Oscar, SnackMasters, Sunkist, VitalChoice

✓ *Frozen "Burger" Options*
- Meat: Applegate hamburger, Great Range bison patties
- Poultry: Applegate turkey burger, Trader Joe's lime turkey burger
- Seafood: Whole Foods wild-caught yellowfin tuna burger, Whole Foods wild-caught mahi mahi burger

✓ **Frozen Breakfast Options**
- Breakfast sausage (2 per serving)
- Brands: Morningstar Farms patty or Veggie Link, Applegate Savory Turkey Breakfast Sausage Link

Vegetarian Proteins

✓ Soy products: tofu, tempeh, soybeans, tofu shirataki noodles
- Brands: NaSoya (lite), Seapoint

✓ Vegetable burgers:
- Brands: Dr. Praeger's California flavor, Gardenburger, Morningstar, Sunshine, Amy's

Produce

Always buy fresh (and seasonal/local when you can)!

Fruit

✓ Fresh fruit: apples, avocado, bananas, blueberries, cantaloupes, cherries, cranberries, grapes, honeydew, kiwi, lemon, lime, nectarine, orange, peach, pear, pineapple, plum, pomegranate (whole or just seeds), prunes, raisins, raspberry, strawberries, tangerines and watermelon

✓ Frozen brands: Sambazon (unsweetened acai), Cascadian Farms (blueberries, raspberries), Wild Harvest (peaches, strawberries)

Vegetables

✓ Fresh vegetables: acorn squash, artichokes, arugula, asparagus, beets, bok choy, broccoli, brussels sprouts, butternut squash, cabbage, carrots, cauliflower, celery, celery root, collard greens, cucumbers, eggplant, endive, ginger, green

beans, Jerusalem artichoke, kabocha squash, kale, kelp, leek, lemon grass, mushrooms, onion, peas, pea shoots, peppers, potatoes, pumpkin, salsify, scallion, shallots, spinach, sweet potatoes, swiss chard, tomatoes, yellow squash and zucchini
- ✓ Frozen brands (all unseasoned): Birds Eye, Cascadian Farm, Seapoint Farms (unsalted, organic), Columbia River Organics (microwave friendly)
- ✓ Canned/jarred vegetables: artichoke hearts, hearts of palm, pumpkin, roasted red peppers
- ✓ Canned/jarred brands: Monterey Farms, Native Forests

Fats

Oils and Vinegars
- ✓ Oils: canola, extra-virgin olive, unfiltered omega-3 olive, grapeseed, peanut, safflower, walnut and toasted sesame
- ✓ Brands: Spectrum (also has sprays), Colavita
- ✓ Vinegars: balsamic, black fig, blood orange, pomegranate, white
- ✓ Brands: Monari Federzoni, Cuisine Perel, Spectrum

Salad Dressings
Balsamic vinegar and a bit of extra-virgin olive oil (or balsamic vinegar and Dijon mustard with a dash of olive oil) is the best route when trying to lose weight, but here are some great salad dressings if you want something with a little flavor.

- ✓ Ingredients to look for: extra virgin olive oil
- ✓ Ingredients to avoid: soybean oil, starches or gums, MSG, potassium osrbate, polysorbate 60, natural and artificial flavors, artifical sweeteners, EDTA, caramel color
- ✓ Brands: Annie's Naturals Organic, Newman's light, Bragg Organic, Gourmet Mist Fusions

Additional Condiments and Spreads
- ✓ Brands: Hellmann's light mayonnaise, Brummel & Brown (yogurt-based butter spread), Sabra and Tribe 100-calorie individually packaged hummus spreads, Desert Pepper Trading company spicy black bean dip, Whole Guacamole

100-calorie guacamole packs, Grey Poupon made with white wine Dijon mustard, 365 organic Dijon mustard, 365 fruit spread, Cucina Antica Tomato Sauces, Hampton Chutney Cilantro Chutney, Le Grand Pesto

Seasonings and Spices
✓ Brands: Whole Foods tequila lime, traditional cajun, thai curry, sesame ginger

Others

Breading Options for Meats
✓ Brands: Hodgson unprocessed bran, Quaker unprocessed bran, Panko bread crumbs, GG Scandinavian Brancrisp Sprinkles, Whole Foods flavored panko bread crumbs

Soups
✓ Ingredients to look for: organic vegetables
✓ Ingredients to avoid: MSG, preservatives, trans fats, soy/corn/ wheat proteins, potassium sorbate, potassium chloride, caramel color, sodium phosphate, calcium chloride, xantham gum
✓ Brands: Health Valley (fat-free and no salt added), Imagine (low sodium), Amy's (light in sodium), Tabatchnick, Fantastic Simmer Soups, Pacific (low sodium)

Protein Shakes and Drinks To-Go
✓ Note: I always prefer food versus drinks, but if you're really in a bind, shakes can be substituted on occasion for breakfast
✓ Brands: Orgain Organic Protein Shake To Go (vanilla and chocolate), Spiru-Tein (1 scoop), Designer Whey Protein (1 scoop)

Frozen Meals
- Kashi
  - » Black Bean Mango, Lime Cilantro Shrimp, Sweet & Sour chicken
- Amy's (many are GF)
  - » Vegetable Lasagne, Mexican Tamale Pie, Spinach Feta in a Pocket Sandwich, Stuffed Pasta Shells, Single-Serve Margherita Pizza

» Light & Lean Pasta & Veggies, Soft Taco Fiesta (any option works)
» Light in Sodium Brown Rice & Vegetables Bowl, Black Bean Enchilada, Single Serve Spinach Pizza
- Organic Bistro (many are GF)
  » Wild Alaskan Salmon, Ginger Chicken, Sesame Ginger Wild Salmon Bowl
- Trader Joe's
  » Reduced Guilt Tilapia with Fava Beans, Reduced Guilt Mac & Cheese, Grilled Eggplant Parmesan, Chicken Tikka Masala
- French Meadow
  » Orange Mango Chicken, Garlic Chicken, Fragrant Curry Chicken
- Ethnic Gourmet
  » Chicken Tikka Marsala
- Sukhi's Indian
  » Vegan Chili
- Evol
  » Teriyaki Chicken Bowl
- Garden Lites
  » Spinach, butternut squash, zucchini, portobello, roasted vegetable

Snacks

Best Afternoon Snack Options under 200 Calories
✓ Savory and crunchy:
- Orville Redenbacher's SmartPop! 100-calorie packs microwave mini bags
- Original all-natural kettle corn, 1 oz bag
- Glenny's Organic Soy Crips (1.3 oz bag or smaller)
- Sea's Gift Roasted Seaweed Snacks (GF and vegan)
- Annie Chun's: Wasabi Seaweed Snacks
- Sabra or Tribe 100-calorie hummus packet (with cut-up veggies or 2 FiberRich crackers)
- Seapoint Farms 100-calorie edamame packets
- Blue Diamond 100-calorie almond packet

✓ Fruit snacks
- Peeled apples
- Kaia Foods Fruit Leather
- Matt's Munchies

✓ Trail mix packets:
- Kopali Organic Mix

✓ Bars:
- Gnu Fiber and Flavor
- Oskyi Fiber Bar
- Go Lean Crunchy!
- Organic Fiber Bar
- Kind (180 or less)
- Luna (mini is also available)
- Luna Protein
- The Simply Bar (GF)
- Cascadian Farm granola bar (2 bars is 1 serving): almond butter flavor
- Males only: Kashi Go Lean Roll, Mojo bar

Sweet After-Dinner Options (Maintenance Only, Everything in Individual Portions):

✓ Cold Treats:
- Edy's slow-churned mini cups
- Skinny Cow mini cups
- Ciao Bella blood orange sorbet pops
- Ciao Bella blood orange sorbet mini cups
- Edy's fruit pops
- Jala ice cream bars
- Arctic Zero ice cream (not individual serving but low cal)

✓ Chocolate cravings:
- Chocolite (chocolate crispy caramel)
- Bissinger's 100-calorie chocolate bar
- Adora dark chocolate calcium
- Kookie Karma Choco Lot
- Sweetriot 100% cacao ribs
- Q.bel wafer rolls

GF = gluten-free

Heather's Acknowledgments

Bread Is the Devil would never have been possible without the help of some talented and thoughtful people.

I want to begin with Kathy Matthews. Kathy, your ability to listen to my words and turn them into useful prose is a true gift. Our ability to collaborate on concepts and the ease with which we worked together was a special pleasure. Your dedication, patience, calmness, positive attitude, and unbelievable stamina made all the difference. You always brought the perfect mix of professionalism and humor to our work sessions, and for that I am forever grateful.

I am indebted to McBride Literary for helping me develop the original concept for the book. Thank you, Margret, for your commitment and for always believing in me.

I am grateful, too, to Andy Barzvi, my literary agent, for taking me under your wing at ICM and helping to make this book a reality.

Thank you to the skillful, hard-working, and energetic team at St. Martin's Press. Kathy Huck, my editor, has been outstanding. Thank you for believing in *Bread Is the Devil* and for your patience and most especially for your helpful edits. Your dedication and attention to details is uncanny and your ideas and creative spin on some of the concepts were marvelous. I also want to thank John Murphy, Nadea Mina, and of course, Sally Richardson. Big thanks as well to all the others at St. Martin's Press on the team from sales, marketing, design, and production.

To my parents, Beth and Nathan Greenbaum, where do I even begin? You gave me the tools that I needed to excel in school and ultimately in life. You filled my childhood with love and support and gave me the confidence I needed to grow and believe in myself. Thank you for all of the inspirational sticky notes, Dad; thank you for always reading to me, Mom; and thank you for telling my first grade teacher that she was wrong, and I *would* go somewhere in life.

I also want to thank my brother and sister, Jordan and Jessica Greenbaum: You two have always driven me to succeed and I am so grateful for all of your support. To my amazing Grandmother Miriam Nickelsporn—ninety years old and one of my greatest advisors in life—I adore you.

To the three mini loves of my life—Zander, Harlan, and Hayes; thank you. You three are my rocks and while our house is total chaos at times, I feel the most peaceful, calm, and happy when we are all together. You three were so amazingly patient this past year, during all those weekends by letting me write away and work long hours. I love you more than you will ever know.

And finally, to all my clients: You are the real inspiration behind this book.

Kathy's Acknowledgments

Writing this book with Heather Bauer has been pure pleasure. She is an absolute delight: incredibly hard-working, remarkably perceptive, and intuitive when it comes to weight loss, and always reliably positive and fun. Margret McBride, agent extraordinaire, got this project out of the gate and I am grateful to her for her friendship and hard work. Andy Barzvi revived this Devil and made the book happen. Kathy Huck, at St. Martin's Press, has been a dedicated and skilled editor, and Heather and I are both grateful for the contributions she made to the final structure and flow of the book. Her assistant, Kate Ottaviano, and the rest of the team at St. Martin's, particularly Sally Richardson and John Murphy, have all proved to be an extraordinary group of dedicated people. It's been a privilege to enjoy their good spirits and enthusiasm for their books and authors. As always, my family, Fred, Greg, and Ted, along with my sister Maggie, have been patient and supportive and I thank them all.

Index